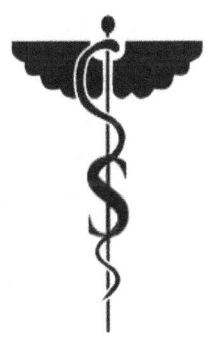

Raymond C. Andrews, M.D.

HOW TO BE A PATIENT
AND
LIVE TO TELL THE TALE!

*A Survival Guide for Today's
Modern Medical Maze*

Other books by Raymond C. Andrews, M.D.

Medical Grail Revised Edition
The Life and Times of Benjamin Wiggins, M.D.
Driving the Great Western Trail in Arizona
Arizona's East-West Trail: A Backcountry Challenge

DVD by Raymond C. Andrews, M.D.

The Great Western Trail in Arizona

Majette Publications First edition 2011
Copyright © 2011-2023 by Raymond C. Andrews, M.D.

www.greatwesterntrailinarizona.com
email: gwtguide@wavecable.com

Cover: Microsoft Clip Art PEO2717 modified by
Raymond C. Andrews, M.D.

ISBN 1456546775
ISBN 978-1456546779

ACKNOWLEDGMENTS

I would like to thank the many patients whose approval of my articles and letters in various publications confirmed the need for this book.

I would especially like to thank Michael J. D'Alto, M.D. , a friend and colleague who graciously volunteered to edit, correct, and suggest changes to make the book more under-standable to the non-professional reader.

TABLE OF CONTENTS

Prologue

Do you remember when you were a child and your parents called old Doc Jones in the middle of the night because you were ill? If you are a young adult you probably don't, since most doctors stopped making house calls before you were born. If you're older, you might recall he arrived at your home, unshaven and grumpy because of the hour. His appearance and gruff manner frightened you initially, but when he gently rested his hand on your belly, your pain and fear disappeared as if by magic.

When your parents asked him how much they owed him for the visit, you heard him answer, "Pay me when you get my bill." You might not have known your father was out of work, but he did, and he never sent his bill.

Today the Doc Joneses in America are almost extinct. A new breed of practitioner has taken their place: the businessman-physician. If *you* call him in the middle of the night because *your* child is ill, he will send you to your local emergency room, even though he knows services there will cost you thousands of dollars and the ED doctor will order many more tests than he would to diagnose your child's illness.

This scene is replayed thousands of times a day across the country, but if you know how the medical system works, you can still find a "Doc Jones" and avoid the financial and physical risks associated with today's treadmill-style medical care.

Historically, doctors cured few diseases and despaired entirely of stemming the plagues that devastated past civilizations. Through persistence and serendipity, however, they learned that the body's most formidable enemies come not from within, but lie in ambush in its environment. These invisible killers include the typhoid fever and hepatitis microbes that contaminate our drinking water, the malaria carrying mosquitoes that live in swampy terrain, and the germs teeming in the excrement collecting in uncovered trenches outside shanty houses.

After centuries of trial and error doctors realized they could prevent these diseases by purifying drinking water, draining swamps, and installing sewers. These simple public health measures defeated our environment's attempts to shorten our existence, which now easily exceeds one hundred years, a life span few attained in earlier times.

Today, space-age machines, such as Computerized Tomography Scanners and Magnetic Resonance Imagers, monitor and measure your health in ways never dreamed of by early doctors. Unfortunately, along with their introduction came the businessman-physician who relies more on what *they* tell him than on what *you* tell him. The reason is obvious: although talking with you is an easier and safer way to arrive at the diagnosis of your disease than is sending you off to have an MRI, it takes time and is less profitable.

In the introduction to the 1979 Surgeon General's report *Healthy People*. Secretary of Health, Education, and Welfare, Joseph Califano at the time declared, "You, the individual, can do more for your own health and well-being than any doctor, any hospital, any drugs, (and) any exotic medical device." I would add that any doctor, any hospital, many drugs and exotic medical devices can do more *dam-*

age to your health in a day than you could ever hope to undo, even with the help of the best malpractice lawyers in the land.

Despite the first dictum of the Hippocratic Oath, *primum non nocere* "first do no harm," many doctors order a battery of laboratory examinations, regardless of their need or danger, before diagnosing even the simplest disease. They call this "defensive medicine," and foolishly believe their patients will not sue them for malpractice if they "perform all the tests."

Competent doctors can easily and inexpensively diagnose almost all of your health problems during your visit to their office. No patient has ever sued his doctor because he correctly diagnosed his disease without ordering a bunch of expensive laboratory tests. He sued when his surgeon amputated his healthy leg instead of the diseased one, and not because he failed to order a test for malaria.

A second, less ethical reason doctors order unnecessary testing is luxury automobiles and alimony payments. These and similar excuses encourage them to do as much as possible to you *before* you recover from your illness on your own, which you will do most of the time. This increases *their* earnings at the same time it increases *your* medical costs, as well as the possibility of permanent injury or death from risky or unnecessary procedures.

This book is the result of years of learning, teaching and the knowledge that the human body is a self-repairing organism that will last many years despite the abuses you heap on it. When it does break down, you should not simply entrust its repairs to anyone bearing a title, no matter how fanciful it may be. *You must actively take part in the decision-making.*

HOW TO BE A PATIENT AND LIVE TO TELL THE TALE! will teach you how to use today's medical system to arrive at the correct diagnosis of your illness or injury while avoiding unnecessary laboratory testing, unwarranted surgical and medical procedures, and dangerous medications *before* they damage your health or drain your budget.

We all will eventually have a serious health problem we hope our doctors will cure. But before we knock on their doors, we will need to know if they are competent and honest and will do their best to resolve our problems quickly and inexpensively, or if they are inept and greedy and will blindly order tests or procedures just to boost their bank deposits. You will also want to know if they will prescribe a proven, safe therapy or a new, expensive, and possibly dangerous medication simply because a drug salesman promised them they would "win" a cruise to the Bahamas if they met a quota.

This book will help you find the Doc Jones in your area. It cannot guarantee you will survive your illness, but it will help you understand what your doctor, pharmacist, and hospital are doing to you, show you how education and skepticism can help you avoid the travails of medical science, and teach you how to make modern medicine work in your favor.

Some of the material in this book may seem unimportant if you receive your care from an HMO or similar organization. If you believe that, you are seriously in error. Ironically, in that case your risk is not *over* treatment, but *under* treatment. Doctors who work for those organizations may not be able to order the care they think you need because their cost-conscious program administrators will not approve expensive therapies.

You should use the information in this book not only to avoid improper care, but also to make sure you receive the correct care.

I do not believe managed care is the solution to our

health care woes, especially since it has moved the profits from doctors' pockets to those of the insurance companies' CEOs. The less of your money they spend on you, the more they can keep for themselves.

Even though it will never happen, I believe if patients paid their own bills, as they did in the "old" days, medical costs would plummet for the following reasons:

1. Patients with minor complaints would stay out of doctor's offices, emergency rooms and hospitals;

2. Patients would shop around for their doctors, choosing the most honest, competent, and reasonably priced. Incompetent doctors would be forced out of practice, and dedicated doctors would again treat the indigent for free;

3. Multi-thousand dollar surgical fees would stop because no one would or could pay them. Surgeons could sue their patients to collect their excessive fees, but they would more likely lower them if they wanted to stay in business.

4. Unnecessary laboratory and other medical costs would plummet for the reasons above.

5. Hospitals would become more competitive since they would have fewer patients. Those who need admission would have checked their charges beforehand, avoiding the more expensive ones. Lest you worry needlessly, expensive care is not superior to inexpensive care, especially since hospitals must follow legal and moral guidelines.

Until such radical ideas become a reality, you will need to understand how the medical system works to safeguard your health and pocketbook.

Chapter One

BET YOUR LIFE:
Understanding the Rules of the Medical Game

"What sort of doctor is he?"
"Well, I don't know much about his ability; but he's got a very good bedside manner."
<u>Punch</u>, March 15, 1884

Before you begin your tour through the medical looking glass, let's see if you know the answers to some of today's most common medical problems. Since your doctor might describe your disease to you as if you were a medical colleague, some of the questions are in "Medicalese." I will show you how to correct this communication problem in a later chapter.

The following quiz will help you identify weaknesses in your patient protection armor.

1. *Primum non nocere* to a physician means:
    a. First collect your fee.
    b. First do no harm.
    c. First order tests "just to be sure."
2. A physician who is not a member of a medical society is incompetent. (T/F)
3. A physician who prescribes the newest medications is more up to date than his colleagues who don't.

(T/F)

4. Physicians are infallible. (T/F)

5. It is a waste of time to ask for a second opinion about your scheduled surgery, as your doctor would never suggest you undergo an unnecessary operation. (T/F)

6. Encourage your doctor to order all the tests he can think of to help diagnose your disease; you would not want him to miss anything important. (T/F)

7. A physician cannot make a correct diagnosis without ordering laboratory studies. (T/F)

8. Arteriograms can be deadly. (T/F)

9. A specialist can diagnose your disease better than a general practitioner. (T/F)

10. The best place to learn about a physician's capabilities is his medical society. (T/F)

11. "Ping-Pong medicine" is:

    a. A TV quiz show for medical interns.

    b. A new Olympic sports competition whereby unethical doctors bounce their patients from one colleague to another to increase their fortunes.

12. Routine laboratory testing will always diagnose your illness. (T/F)

13. Differential diagnosis (where different diseases could be the cause of your symptoms) is one reason for excessive laboratory testing. (T/F)

14. Skin testing is a safe way to find out if you are allergic to a medication. (T/F)

15. If surgeon is Board Certified, he is qualified to perform your operation. (T/F)

16. All doctors are geniuses, so you do not need to describe your problem to them. They will know what is wrong with you by simply looking into your charming blue eyes. (T/F)

17. Aspirin and vitamins are not real medications and you may safely take as many as you like. (T/F)
18. Expensive therapies and treatments are more often unnecessary than inexpensive prescriptions. (T/F)
19. Doctors should routinely perform a cardiac angiogram to complete your work-up for *angina pectoris*. (T/F)
20. If you have had heart surgery to stop your chest pain, you don't need to quit smoking. (T/F)
21. The *Physicians' Desk Reference* (now the Internet) is a good place to find out if the primary use of your medication is to treat your health problem. (T/F)
22. If a mother says her child is ill and a pediatrician says he isn't, the pediatrician is right. (T/F)
23. Your doctor can best treat fever without other symptoms with an antibiotic, which he must prescribe if it does not disappear in two days. (T/F)
24. If a new symptom occurs after starting drug therapy:
    a. You must presume it to be due to the medication until proven otherwise.
    b. Your doctor should treat it immediately with another medication before it worsens.
    c. It means your disease is worsening, and you should make sure your will is up-to-date.
25. The newest medications are always more effective than older ones. (T/F)
26. If one pill is good for you, five will be even better. (T/F)
27. Always ask your doctor for an injection instead of pills. This way you won't have to wake up during the night to take your medication. (T/F)
28. Vitamins, like Wonder bread, build bodies 189 ways, so take as many as you can as often as you

can. (T/F)

29. Save your left over medication since you may need it again. (T/F)

30. Sleeping pills:

    a. Are safe to take for long periods of time.

    b. Should never be prescribed for the elderly.

    c. Are hard to find in drugstores nowadays since they are not profitable for pharmaceutical houses.

31. All medications have side effects. (T/F)

32. You pay a doctor for his prescription. If he does not give you one at the end of your visit, he is not a good doctor. (T/F)

33. Ask your doctor about the side effects of the medication he prescribes. Knowing what they are may keep you from taking them. (T/F)

34. Because of intensive research in pharmaceutical laboratories, few new drugs are dangerous. (T/F)

35. People have used aspirin to commit suicide. (T/F)

36. Patients hospitalized for unrecognized drug reactions:

    a. Do not exist.

    b. May account for as much as 20% of the total hospital population.

    c. Only occur if their doctors are out of town and their substitutes are fresh out of medical school and still have a lot to learn.

37. Pharmaceutical houses are too ethically correct to offer rewards to doctors that prescribe their medications. (T/F)

38. Drug companies sell identical drugs under different names to help doctors prescribe a "new medication" for their uninformed patients. (T/F)

39. If your prescription allows you to decide the dosage and frequency of your medication, always take the

maximum prescribed, and maybe a little more. It will help you get well sooner. (T/F)

40. Medications do not cross the placenta blood barrier, so it's safe to take them during pregnancy. This includes nicotine and alcohol. (T/F)

41. Modern medications are safer than the chemically impure drugs of earlier times. (T/F)

42. Hyperactive children need heavy sedation so they don't hurt themselves while playing in the school-yard. (T/F)

43. Therapy is not opinion. Doctors must adhere to standardized tables when prescribing medication in order not to harm their patients. (T/F)

44. If you could choose someone to treat your uncom-plicated flu, it would be:
    a. A lung specialist.
    b. Grandma.
    c. Soupy Sales.

45. It is a good idea for your doctor to hospitalize you during any illness, since he can order all your labo-ratory tests more conveniently for you. (T/F)

46. Doctors hospitalize patients only when necessary. (T/F)

47. Never check your medical bills. Computers compile them and therefore are correct. (T/F)

48. Government rules fix hospital prices, so there is no need to shop around for lower prices. (T/F)

49. There is an increase in patient mortality when doc-tors in socialized countries strike for higher wages. (T/F)

50. Dying at home is un-American and a violation of the Human Rights Act. (T/F)

51. Modern, expensive, obstetrical monitoring equip-ment guarantees your unborn child will be physi-

cally, mentally, and emotionally superior to one born in a taxicab for $8.95 plus tip. (T/F)

52. An $80.00 chest X-ray is more accurate than one that costs $40.00. (T/F)

53. If your doctor is away, the best place to get care is in your local emergency room. (T/F)

54. Emergency rooms are the same everywhere, so you can be sure the one nearest you will be able to treat even your most serious problem. (T/F)

55. If your local hospital administrator tells you he has a neurosurgeon on his staff, you can be sure he will be immediately available when you need him. (T/F)

56. A moonlighter in the emergency room may be:
a. A doctor who dedicates his time to helping the needy for free.
b. A doctor not trained in emergency medicine, but who needs extra money to support his family.
c. A drunk who performs an obscene gesture in the ED.

57. Every admission from an emergency room to a hospital's main wards is necessary. (T/F)

58. Medicenters are more efficient than traditional doctor's office. (T/F)

59. State certification guarantees that your doctor knows how to use his office X-ray machine correctly. (T/F)

60. Kickbacks are unknown in medicine. You can be certain that any test your doctor orders and is performed in a private laboratory will be in your best interests. (T/F)

61. A reputable laboratory will charge less than a hospital would for the same services. (T/F)

62. A doctor will never hospitalize an uninsured patient just to perform simple laboratory tests. (T/F)

63. All hospitals charge the same fee for the same test performed by the same technician on an outpatient, an inpatient, or a patient who arrives to the hospital late at night. (T/F)

64. It's useless to try to get your money back if your health care provider overcharged you. (T/F)

65. Doctors can prevent few diseases. (T/F)

66. Seven to 12% of all laboratory reports are wrong. (T/F)

67. It is a false sense of security if you believe you are in perfect health after your doctor tells you "all your tests are normal." (T/F)

68. If you are a healthy, vigorous person with no symptoms of illness, you do not need a yearly physical, since the likelihood of uncovering an unsuspected disease is almost nonexistent. (T/F)

69. Even if you had a physical a month ago, you should not rely on its glowing results as proof your new chest pain is unimportant, nor should you wait until your next physical before seeking advice. (T/F)

70. One problem with the Measles, Mumps, and Rubella vaccine is that up to 25% of children vaccinated with it may still develop those diseases, or an atypical form of them, which will present diagnostic difficulties for the children's doctors. (T/F)

71. Healthy young adults should not receive the influenza vaccine. (T/F)

72. A yearly electrocardiogram will prevent you from dying of a heart attack. (T/F)

73. Your blood pressure may rise when you are nervous. (T/F)

74. If most of your 30 blood tests are abnormal, you are too. If only one is, as a rule you are not. (T/F)

75. Personally review your test results and/or request a

written summary of them. Under no condition accept your doctor's promise, "If you do not hear from me, it means the tests are normal." (T/F)

Answers	1-B	2-F	3-F
4-F	5-F	6-F	7-F
8-T	9-F	10-F	11-C
12-F	13-T	14-F	15-F
16-F	17-F	18-T	19-F
20-F	21-T	22-F	23-F
24-A	25-F	26-F	27-F
28-F	29-F	30-B	31-T
32-F	33-T	34-F	35-T
36-B	37-F	38-T	39-F
40-F	41-F	42-F	43-F
44-B	45-F	46-F	47-F
48-F	49-F	50-F	51-F
52-F	53-F	54-F	55-F
56-B	57-F	58-F	59-F
60-F	61-T	62-T	63-F
64-F	65-T	66-T	67-T
68-T	69-T	70-T	71-T
72-F	73-T	74-T	75-T

EVALUATION OF RESPONSES

Less than five errors.

Congratulations! Your score guarantees you will recognize a competent doctor when you see one, "consume" only the health care you need, and keep your house and other possessions if you survive your illness and its treatment. (This book does not offer miracles, such as modification of inherited diseases that negatively influence longevity. See your local shaman for help in that field.)

You also might qualify as a director of your local health-consumer protection agency.

Five to fifteen errors:

Take Grandma with you to the doctor for any serious medical problems, and avoid all non urgent confrontations with a health-care provider. On days when your horoscope suggests risk of injury or contagion, lock yourself in your bedroom until the stars again twinkle in your favor.

Fifteen to twenty-five errors:

Pay your insurance premiums and transfer all your personal possessions to a healthy pet that will allow you unrestricted use of them during your brief lifetime.

More than twenty-five errors:

I never intended this book to be a simple table adornment. I suggest you read it and retake the test. It may surprise you to learn that a dog-eared book is a *real* conversation piece.

Aide-toi, le ciel t'aidera! "Help yourself, and heaven will help you!"

Chapter Two

WIN THE LOTTERY:
Choosing Your Ideal Doctor

"Life is short, the art long, opportunity fleeting, experiment treacherous, judgment difficult."
Hippocrates

Today's space-age medical technology has fewer healing powers than the comforting arm your doctor drapes over your shoulders while he tells you that you don't need tests or medications, and assures you that you will get well on your own in a day or two. As most diseases resolve by themselves in a brief period of time, his gesture is humane but unprofitable. If he suggests you return to see him in four days *only* if you are still sick, he will lose the income from your return visit "just to see how you are doing," as well as whatever he would have earned from the testing and therapy he could have performed at your initial visit.

Doctors know that "the most common disease is the most common." This means that fever and cough in January in America are usually symptoms of the flu and not of Bubonic plague. Keep this in mind before you visit a doctor for your cough and fever next winter. Go if you must, but statistically, your illness will be minor and fleeting. To avoid unnecessary expense and medication, you must go to a doctor who won't treat your fever as a symptom of an exotic disease.

Your Search for the Ideal Physician

When I was an intern many years ago, every evening Mary, an elderly patient with severe heart disease, went into pulmonary edema (her lungs filled with water) when another intern was on duty. Yet she slept peacefully through the night when I or another intern was on call. The care she received from each of us was identical, but as she told me, she had no confidence in Dr. X. Whenever he was on duty her apprehension and adrenaline levels were more than her tired heart could cope with, and it failed.

Confidence in your doctor's abilities is important, but you should not allow him unbridled control over your health or pocketbook simply because of his good bedside manner.

So how do you find a competent doctor you can trust? First, you need a list of all the doctors in your area that treat your problem. You'll find it in your phone book's yellow pages (yes, they are still around) or online. Hospitals and medical societies will supply you with lists of the names of their members. These lists will not be identical, since a doctor does not need to be a member of a medical society to work in a hospital. If you go to an emergency room for care, before you leave, hospital personnel will give you a list of their doctors on call who must offer you follow-up treatment if you do not have a doctor of your own.

These are lists of doctors you will still need to evaluate, since hospitals and medical societies will not tell you if their doctors are competent or if they overcharge their patients. Nor will they tell you if they have been sued for malpractice or have been the subject of patient or insurance company complaints, although you may be able to discover this information from state licensing websites. Lastly, they will refer you only to members of their respective groups since it is in their best interest to do so. A hospital's representative would never refer you to a doctor who works in another hospital, since he (also refers to "he/she" in this book) would lose your future business. And if you ask him about one who is not on his list, he will tell you he never heard of him, but "why not try our Dr. X, a well-known specialist?"

The American Medical Association has created a website (http://www.ama-assn.org/) for patients to find a "perfect match" for their medical needs. The organization's Doctor Finder service is well-intentioned but self-serving. On the site it warns: "Make sure the doctor you choose supports quality patient care and the future of our nation's health. Choose an AMA-member physician or encourage your non-member to join the AMA today."

Since I have never met a doctor who did not support quality health care and the future of our nation's health, every doctor qualifies. Instead of that notice, I would have preferred to read: "Make sure your physician is competent, honest and caring." These qualities are much more important to you than his political affiliations.

The AMA's member doctors in theory must have proper credentials, meet ethical standards, and properly run their offices. Patient satisfaction and clinical performance are important, but I doubt the AMA will withhold accreditation from doctors who routinely order unnecessary tests and medications just to make you feel he's doing his job. Those barred from practice and membership in any society or hospital usually have drug or alcohol addictions, have committed acts of malpractice that defy logic, have preyed sexually on patients of any age or sex, or have committed insurance fraud.

An online listing of doctors will not necessarily help you find one to fit your needs, although it will give you a list of names to evaluate as well as some you need to avoid. State medical societies offer physician information at their websites, such as where they went to school, their specialty, their office location, if their license is current, and if there are criminal convictions or disciplinary actions against them.

All this information is helpful, but you still need to independently evaluate their doctors. A medical society is simply a social club that is no more prestigious than any other self-serving group. Do not let the fancy titles it awards its members influence your choice. Its "committee president for the evaluation of the effect of postage stamp mucilage on stuttering" may be a good choice if you like to lick postage stamps and stutter, but he may not be the one to cure your migraine headache. You don't want a politician-physician who spends all his time in meetings. You want one who spends his time in medicine's trenches.

Board certification is a qualification that adds a few more letters to a doctor's title, and you need to understand what they are. A boarded physician is one who has had training beyond an internship and has taken an examination to qualify him as a specialist in a particular field, such as neurosurgery or obstetrics. You can find a list of bona fide boards recognized by the American Board of Medical Specialties at http://www.abms.org/. Each has its own requirements, but three or four years of training followed by a comprehensive examination usually satisfy most of them.

Practitioners of the noble art have never lacked ingenuity, and at least 115 lesser, self-designated boards are also on the scene for those who do not qualify for the traditional ones. Many state medical boards and the American Board of Medical Specialties do not recognize them, and you should consider their members with caution.

The directory published by the American Board of Medical Specialties is in public libraries and on the Internet. Here you will also find a listing of a doctor's credentials.

A doctor who does not have hospital privileges, is not a member of the AMA, and is not board certified, is not necessarily incompetent. You should check into his background thoroughly, but do not exclude him from consideration simply because he is not on someone's list. A competent general practice doctor can treat most of your ailments in his office just as competently as a board certified family practice doctor can, and will refer you to a colleague if you are seriously ill and need hospitalization that he cannot provide.

This doctor can be a good choice. Since he often does not have patients in the hospital, your appointments with him will likely be on time, he will not run off to the ED in the middle of your pap smear to treat an emergency, and his rates may be lower for the same services.

It is important to understand that a doctor is not competent simply because he is on the staff of a certain hospital, or incompetent because he is not, although a neurosurgeon who offers to remove your brain tumor in a Motel 6 probably has a past you need to know about before you consent to surgery.

A competent and capable doctor who does not have malpractice insurance cannot work in a hospital. This is because the law can force anyone even remotely related to an act of malpractice to pay the damages if the perpetrator cannot. Simply put, since a hospital does not want to pay out millions for the uninsured doctor who cut off your good leg instead of your gangrenous one, he will not allow him to work in its institution.

Lawyers with the Willie Sutton philosophy perpetuate this state of affairs. When someone asked Willie why he robbed banks, he answered, "Because that's where the money is." A lawyer will not sue the uninsured doctor who cut off your good leg because he knows his client will not win enough in court to cover his fees. But if he sues your surgeon's colleagues, the nurses, and the hospital, their insurance companies will settle out of court for large sums of money, even if their clients are innocent, simply to cut legal costs and to avoid the possibility of even higher jury awards.

Years ago a patient who did not follow my written instructions had an allergic reaction to the medication I had prescribed for her, and sued me. My insurance company looked into her complaint and stated in writing that a panel of specialists had determined that my diagnosis, therapy, and advice had been correct, and that the woman herself was at fault because she had not followed the written advice I had given her. It added that if I would sign a release, it would pay the woman the sum she had sought at no cost to me. I politely told the company that since my care was correct, I would sue both it and the woman if they paid her even a dime of her unjustified request.

Episodes like this are one reason medical care is so costly. I would not have had to pay the woman out-of-pocket, but my malpractice insurance cost would have increased the following year, and I would have had to raise my patient fees to cover my increased overhead. We all pay for the bill for those patients who refuse to accept responsibility for their own care, as well as for those ambulance-chasing lawyers who let their clients live their dishonest dream because they themselves profit from it.

Madison Avenue Physicians

Whether to advertise or not is an animated point of discussion among today's businessmen-physicians, but is it possible to advertise honesty, competence, or compassion? I do not think so. Word of mouth is still the best way to learn about a doctor's merits, and your pharmacist and neighbors are good sources of information about the practitioners in your community. A few minutes' conversation with any of them should be enough to help you find a doctor suitable for your needs.

Questions to ask them include: Is his receptionist efficient and professional, or does she yell your information to her doctor over a tin can and waxed string communications center in the waiting room for everypne there to hear?

HIPAA rules guarantee privacy, but they are not retroactive. (http://en.wikipedia.org/wiki/Health_Insurance_Portability_ and_Accountability_Act)

Also, beware of the nurse who assumes the role of diagnostician ("Got an ulcer out here, Doc."). A nurse is not a doctor, and it may take more experience than she has to arrive at a correct diagnosis or to understand the severity of certain symptoms. A tragic example is that of an elderly man with severe headache, nausea, vomiting, and a blood pressure of 330/180 mm Hg. who called his doctor near his office's closing time. The nurse who received the call did not relay *all* the patient's symptoms to the doctor as he hurried out the door. Because of poor communication, his inappropriate advice was to "take two Valium tablets and call me in the morning." That night the patient died of a ruptured brain aneurysm, and the next morning his family's lawyer called him in the deceased's stead.

Next you will need to know if the doctor you're considering examines his patients himself, or if he just "pills 'em and pushes 'em" without rising from his desk. It is also important to know if his physician assistant examines you, and he just parrots his diagnosis. Usually this is acceptable, but not if the assistant thinks your stomach pain is due to something you ate and not the leaking aortic aneurysm that will kill you.

Method of Payment

You will also want to know if the doctor's primary concern is your health or your insurance policy, since an insured patient will undergo more complicated, unnecessary examinations and treatments than an uninsured patient. You might not realize an insurance hunter is victimizing you, but if a doctor orders a battery of tests even before he examines you, he is. More about this later, but for now, know that economic disaster or worse may await you if you check the wrong "insured status" box on your chart.

Will he treat you if you do not have money to pay him at the time of your visit? Maybe not, in fact his secretary may not even give you an appointment if she suspects you will not be able to pay your bill. But if you suddenly feel deathly ill, drop into a doctor's office unannounced, and he refuses to help you because you can't pay him for his services, it is a serious crime. Since it will bring government lawyers into town in a hurry, a doctor needs to be certain that you will not face severe complications or death before you reach your new destination. Nevertheless, illnesses do not always occur on paydays, and it will be comforting to know beforehand that your credit is good.

You will also need to know about his charges; are they high compared to other doctors? Will he order laboratory tests each time you enter his office? Even if he advertises that testing in his office costs half of what it does elsewhere, the costs of his obligatory testing will make your bill higher than if you had gone to a competent doctor who charges more for the visit, but orders laboratory tests only when you need them.

Does his treatment routinely include a costly injection? Does he demand a follow-up visit even for minor illnesses and injuries? And finally, does he see his patients close to their scheduled times, or does he make them idle for hours in his waiting room? You may allow some leeway on this last point since emergencies do disrupt office schedules, and patients who thought they had minor problems sometimes need more time than was originally allotted them. However, if your doctor arrives late with a golf bag slung over his shoulder, move on.

Next, ask your pharmacist which doctor prescribes the *fewest* medications. This information may not be good for his business, but it will be good for you. Also, ask him which doctor always prescribes the newest drugs on the market. A doctor who always prescribes the newest drug releases may seem to be up-to-date, but avoid him. Drug companies hide the unpleasant side effects of their newest drugs in complicated statistics, and their price is many times greater than older, safer medications. Simple blood thinners, of which aspirin is the last expensive and most common, now cost up to $8,000.00 per year.

Tell the pharmacist you do not want to take unnecessary, outrageously priced medication, prescribed or not, but because of his help in selecting a doctor that fits the above description, you will patronize his shop. Many pharmacies today are located in super stores, so you can easily keep this promise by shopping for other items while your prescription is being filled.

It will be difficult to find a doctor who will fulfill all of your financial, emotional, and health needs, but the devil you know is better than the one you don't. You may not mind the expense of a urine test at each visit if your doctor satisfies your other needs. Neither might you mind waiting long hours if you are poor and know he will charge you according to your ability to pay.

Your First Appointment

After finding a doctor you feel may serve your needs, ask him for a free introductory appointment. It is important to meet the person who may someday decide whether you live or die following an accident or severe illness. Most doctors will be happy to meet with you for a few minutes to decide if there is a basis for a continuing relationship. You might even like to know that his shoulder length hair hides tattoos running down his neck and three diamond rings in his left earlobe. If you feel uncomfortable with a heavy metal doctor, move on to your next candidate.

You should also ask him if he's read any good books lately. Dartmouth and other medical schools are implementing "Literature and Medicine" courses to teach their students compassion. If they succeed, we may again have doctors who understand there is more to patients than their symptoms and insurance status. Since compassion is far more curative than pills in treating many diseases, your patient-doctor relationship would also improve.

Warning Bells

During your early office visits, any of the following suggestions should warn you to reconsider your choice of doctor:

1. "I would like to perform a few tests."

I will discuss what laboratory tests can do for or to you in a later chapter, but for the moment all you need to know is that you must verify the need for all tests or procedures your physician requests before having them done. You shouldn't refuse testing under urgent or emergency conditions as it may save your life, but physicians do not order tests only in emergencies. If you have doubts, to avoid unnecessary tests, invent an excuse why you have to wait for several weeks before getting them done.

A seriously ill relative in a distant part of the country is a good reason to leave town urgently. Another is a long planned-for vacation. If your physician agrees to wait until you return from your cruise in the Bahamas, you do not need the tests.

If you really do need to have a test done, it should be performed as soon as possible. A patient with a failing heart should have an electrocardiogram (ECG) and other cardiac function tests performed *immediately*. Similar examinations performed on a champion cross-country skier with heartburn are unnecessary and can be postponed indefinitely.

If your doctor orders a chest X-ray and an electrocardiogram for your low back pain, you have fallen into the "routine test" trap. Your doctor may be incompetent, greedy, or because he felt the real purpose of your visit was to sue him, so he ordered those useless examinations in the mistaken belief they will prevent future legal problems. No matter what his reason, this would be a good time to change doctors.

If you are unquestionably ill and if the test results do not show the cause, a real problem exists. You have again fallen into the "routine test" trap, but this time it is much more serious because your doctor is fishing for a diagnosis. He has no idea what is causing your problem, and he is blindly ordering test after test, hoping his laboratory or a radiologist will make the diagnosis for him.

If he knew what was ailing you, he would have ordered the *correct* test to *confirm* his diagnosis. In this case the explanation, "I've performed all the tests and can find nothing wrong," is unacceptable. If your symptoms persist and you are still worried about them, now is another good time to change doctors.

2. "There are several possible causes for your symptoms."

In medicine there is a demon called "differential diagnosis." This means your doctor cannot suspect a kidney stone as the sole cause of the severe pain in your left side that travels down to your lower belly. Even though a simple urine test will usually confirm this diagnosis, because of the rules of differential diagnosis, he must consider your pancreas and heart as possible causes, since these are also on the left side of your body. If you are female, he may also think about a tubal pregnancy as well as the rare situs inversus, which flips your internal organs and places your appendix on your left side.

A competent doctor will perform a differential diagnosis in his head, eliminating the unlikely causes and ascribing all your symptoms to one disease he can then confirm with a single test. He will never order a dozen tests to exclude all the other diseases that have only one symptom in common with yours.

If your doctor is pressuring you to undergo multiple testing, you can decrease your costs and help him improve his diagnostic skills by asking him which *specific* disease he thinks you have. He should offer *one* diagnosis. If he does but still proposes a battery of tests, ask him if there is *one* test that will confirm his diagnosis. If there is, have him order it.

If he suggests more than one diagnosis, ask him to explain why. There will be times when he will legitimately suspect more than one cause for your illness. However, if after testing he still comes up with five diagnoses, one for each of your symptoms, believe none of them. If you enjoy watching people squirm, tell him that Dr. Osler, a brilliant diagnostician from the 19th Century, believed a doctor who needed two diagnoses to explain the same symptoms would be wrong half the time.

If your doctor can arrive at a diagnosis only after ordering a battery of tests each time you are ill, you have made a poor choice and should start your search anew.

3. "Let me give you a shot."

What your physician may mean here is, "Help me increase my bank balance." You can take most medications by mouth, although vaccinations, insulin, and allergy desensitizing serums are examples of injectable only medications. There are others, but the shot doctors distinguish themselves by giving injections to *all* their patients at each office visit without regard to urgency, need, or severity of their disease.

Shun them, if only to avoid a severe or fatal allergic drug reaction. This is even more important if you have had a reaction to an injection in the past. The scratch, conjunctival, and intradermal tests with dilute solutions of a medication, which your doctor may suggest as a means to confirm or exclude your allergy, are unreliable and not without hazard.

If you don't want an injection and don't feel ill, ask your doctor if his medication exists in pill form and have him prescribe it. If he offers you a prescription *and* a shot just to help you recover more quickly, tell him a doctor once gave you an injection and you almost died from shock. If he tells you his injection is not an antibiotic and will not cause a problem, your final response as you walk out of his office for the last time, should be that your reaction was to the ingredient used to dissolve the medication and all injectable medications contain it.

4. "Take all these pills."

Most diseases resolve on their own without medication, although your doctor may prescribe a drug to decrease annoying symptoms while they do. For example, cough syrups control the respiratory symptoms of the flu and aspirin relieves the pain of a sprained ankle, yet both of these problems will resolve completely without medication. Problems arise when a doctor prescribes penicillin for the flu and injects cortisone into your ligaments for the strain. Both are inappropriate and can cause a great deal of unpleasantness.

You may need to take medication for extended periods to combat common illnesses, such as diabetes, hypertension, and arthritis. Usually a doctor will prescribe drugs for these diseases only if they do not respond to weight control, diet, exercise, improved mental outlook, or the abolition of bad habits, such as drinking, smoking, and drug abuse. If he does, follow his orders.

However, *all* medications have side effects, sometimes mild and sometimes deadly. If they are unnecessary or inappropriate for your illness, do not take them.

5. "You need an operation."

Never risk your life undergoing an unnecessary operation! A surgeon will not suggest unnecessary surgery if *you have no insurance,* and neither will a physician who will not gain financially even if you do. If drastic therapy is suggested, be certain there is no other method of treating your problem before agreeing to it. I will explain how to do this in a later chapter. For now know that even earnest doctors may not know all the latest therapies and techniques, and that you should always get a second opinion.

Second Opinions

Before consenting to any non-emergency operation, *always* get a second opinion. Insurance companies recommend them to reduce unnecessary surgery, and incidentally their costs. They have statistics to show this works. Doctors have statistics to show it does not.

A second opinion *is* a valid way to find out if you need surgery, but fails in its purpose if a doctor who wants to operate refers you to his partner. In this case, the second opinion will mirror the first, resulting only in higher medical costs and no benefit to you.

For example, you should get a second opinion before beginning treatment for *hyper*thyroidism. In this disease the thyroid gland in your neck turns up your body's thermostat, causing weight loss, sweating, weakness, heat intolerance, and a fast heartbeat.

To treat this disease, a surgeon will remove part of your gland. This will reduce the amount of hormone it releases into your blood stream, and thus relieve your symptoms. If your thyroid is producing twice as much hormone than it should, half of it will produce only half as much, or an amount equal to that of a normal gland.

It is logical, but no surgeon knows exactly how much of the gland to remove. If he removes too much, *hypo*thyroidism will result, with symptoms of weight gain, weakness, and cold intolerance. If he removes too little, you will improve but you will continue to have the same symptoms you had before your surgery.

You can predict what treatment the surgeon's partner will suggest if you ask him for a second opinion.

If you ask a radiologist, he might suggest radioactive iodine. What is the result of his therapy? The possibility of developing hypothyroidism, thyroid cancer later in life, and damage to your genetic pool. If you are pregnant, this therapy is not for you. But if you choose it, at least you will not have a scar on your neck for the entire world to see.

Last, if you ask an endocrinologist or your family doctor, they would likely suggest medication in pill form. They can check its effectiveness with blood tests and by the simple question: "How do you feel today?"

Therapy is Opinion

Chiropractors, acupuncturists, macrobiologists, and other proponents of alternative medicine have differing opinions about the cause and treatments of the same diseases. Even when orthodox physicians agree on the diagnosis, therapy is still opinion, and there are many treatment choices for any disease.

Therefore, each generalist or specialist will favor the therapy he knows best and discriminate against those of his colleagues. To get maximum benefit from the system, especially if the proposed therapy is dangerous, seek a second opinion from an internist or general practitioner who is *not* associated with the doctor who proposed the original therapy. If non-urgent surgery was suggested, search out a doctor who does *not operate* nor *assist* at surgery, and who practices away from your general area.

As a fail-safe, tell your out-of-town doctor you want only his opinion about a therapy proposed by a nameless colleague, and that he will not take part in your treatment program. The universal implementation of digital record keeping by insurance companies today has made it easy for your medical history to travel instantaneously between doctors. To avoid this, refuse access to your records to this consultant when you fill out the questionnaire regarding the reason for your visit to his office.

Later you can switch to your his care if you like his manner and professionalism, but do not tell him this at the time of your visit since it would nullify its purpose. If he knows he will not be involved in your care, he will likely give you an honest opinion, especially if you can subtly make him understand your attorney might want to talk with him if complications result from a therapy he approves but which is later determined to be unnecessary.

He will make "Honest Abe" look like a piker.

Surgeons

Never go to a surgeon for a second opinion about surgery, since he earns his income by operating on disembodied organs ("I've got a gall-bladder in an hour.") Even if he believed a salve or pill would solve your problem, he would not prescribe it until *after* he performed your surgery.

According to statistics, there are too many surgeons, performing too much surgery, with too little expertise, on too many patients. The certificate on their office walls testifies only to the fact they have completed their residencies;

it does not guarantee they are technically efficient or up-to-date. If you need heart surgery and the surgeon you're referred to performs it only once a year, your odds of survival are better *without* the surgery and *with* your disease.

The more times a surgeon performs an operation, the more skillful he will be. If you suspect your surgeon spends more time on his yacht than in the operating suite, politely refuse his offer for an appendix transplant and head straight for the nearest major medical center where other surgeons perform the operation many times a day.

One operation every few months is not enough to keep him proficient, and if he is the only one performing the operation in his hospital, the ancillary personnel will not be proficient either. Since you will spend your recovery with nurses, technicians, and doctors' assistants, their experience is tantamount to your survival.

Since it costs no more to get the best medical care, evaluate all the possibilities before undergoing any permanent or dangerous treatment.

As a final note, the President's Advisory Commission on Consumer Protection and Quality in the Health Care Industry adopted a "Consumer Bill of Rights and Responsibilities" in 1998. Many health plans have adopted these principles, and since you need to know you have a say in your care, I list some of them here. I also include what I believe to be your obligations, since any contract involves at least two parties.

1. Consumers have the right to receive accurate, easily understood information and help in making informed health-care decisions about their health plans, providers and facilities.

Obligation: to request and to study all the information available to you before agreeing to any test or treatment.

2. Consumers have the right to a choice of health care

providers sufficient to assure access to appropriate high-quality health care.

Obligation: to evaluate thoroughly any doctor whom you consider to be a possible provider of your care. Just because his name appears on an HMO roster does not mean that he is automatically competent and caring.

3. Consumers have the right to access emergency health care services when and where the need arises. Health plans should provide payment when a consumer presents to an emergency department with acute symptoms of sufficient severity, including severe pain – such that a prudent "layperson" could reasonably expect the absence of medical attention to result in placing the consumer's health in serious jeopardy, serious injury to bodily functions, or serious dysfunction of any bodily organ or part.

Obligation: to not misuse your local emergency room by going there for the minor ills and ailments you should know how to treat at home.

4. Consumers have the right and responsibility to fully take part in all decisions related to their medical care. Consumers who are unable to fully participate in treatment decisions have the right to be represented by parents, guardians, family members, or other conservators.

Obligation: to participate effectively in your care, you must be informed. If you do not ask questions, you will not understand the material presented to you. If your provider explains his plans in words you do not understand, ask him to speak your language. You cannot make a valid decision if you cannot understand what is being offered.

5. Consumers have the right to considerate, respectful care from all members of the health care industry at all times and under all circumstances. An environment of mutual respect is essential to maintain a quality health care system.

Consumers must not be discriminated against in the delivery of health care services consistent with the benefits covered in their policy, or as required by law, based on race, ethnicity, national origin, religion, sex, age, mental or physical disability, sexual orientation, genetic information, or source of payment,

Consumers who are eligible for coverage under the terms and conditions of a health plan or program, or as required by law, must not be discriminated against in marketing and enrollment practices based on race, ethnicity, national origin, religion, sex, age, mental or physical disability, sexual orientation, genetic information, or source of payment.

Obligation: to treat medical personnel as you wish them to treat you. If your provider thinks you do not need an antibiotic for the flu, it is not because you are brown, green, or because you speak in an incomprehensible dialect from an uncharted island in the Pacific. It is because you don't need it. Accept his opinion or calmly question it.

6. Consumers have the right to communicate with health care providers in confidence and to have the confidentiality of their individually identifiable health care information protected. Consumers also have the right to review and copy their own medical records and request amendments to their records.

Obligation: Say "please" and "thank you," and offer to pay for the copies. You probably won't have to, but it's a nice gesture.

7. All consumers have the right to a fair and efficient process for resolving differences with their health plans, health care providers, and the institutions that serve them, including a rigorous system of internal review and an independent system of external review.

Obligation: You must ask what the procedure is, and

follow it precisely. Grumbling to your friends about your supposed inequity will not solve your problem.

None of these rights guarantees your doctor will correctly diagnose your ailment, will perform only necessary tests, or will prescribe the right medication to treat your disease. They do guarantee you will be treated humanely during your illness.

Chapter Three

TOUR THE INNER SANCTUM:
Discovering What Goes on behind the Door of Your
Doctor's Office

"I suppose one has a greater sense of intel-
lectual degradation after an interview with a
doctor than from any human experience."
Alice James (1848–92), U.S. diarist.

Since my purpose in writing this book is to teach you
how to survive physically and economically when you need
medical care, the following guide will help you determine
whether your doctor is needlessly endangering your health
or exhausting your budget.

Medicine is a business. If you doubt that, try to make
an appointment with a doctor without first showing his
billing clerk your insurance card or prepaying your estimated charges. It is more common nowadays for a doctor
to demand prepayment for his services than it was years
ago, but there are still practitioners who will bill you after
your visit and accept monthly payments if necessary. If
your doctor demands to be paid first, he is obviously much
more interested in his economic welfare than in yours, and
I suggest you find one who is less mercenary.

Once you have passed the main desk, your trip into the

world of medicine will vary according to local custom. A nurse may escort you fully dressed into a consultation room where your doctor will discuss your problem with you, or she may ask you to undress and wait in an examining room for a combined questioning and examining session. The latter occurs because it is quicker if your problem is obvious or needs immediate treatment.

In either case, your visit must include at least two parts: the history of your disease and your physical examination. I will describe a third, laboratory testing, in a later chapter.

The single most important part of your entire examination is what you tell your doctor. You can't just drop off your body with a note, "Please fix." You need to tell him exactly what is wrong with you, and you will do that in the "history" of your illness. This is where you explain in English what your doctor will record on your chart in unreadable Medicalese. It may be as simple as, "I cut my finger." How you did it may be important, but since your problem is obvious, your doctor can treat it even if you don't tell him you were trying to open a can of beans with a table saw.

If you have a chronic or worsening problem, however, a *complete* history is necessary. A competent doctor can diagnose most of your diseases simply by talking with you, but if he orders a bunch of tests without first asking you a single question, he will probably misdiagnose your illness.

The history contains subheadings that may vary from the order below. Your doctor may skip it entirely if you have an ingrown toenail or something similarly obvious, but not if your problem is serious or obscure.

The standard divisions of the history are the:
1. Chief Complaint
2. Present Illness
3. Family History

4. <u>Past History</u>
5. <u>Personal History</u>
6. <u>Social History</u>
7. <u>Review of Systems</u>

Your Chief Complaint

Your doctor needs to know why you have come to see him. You can talk to him alone if you can remember the details of your problem, or if it is too personal to share with the neighbor or relative that accompanied you to his office. A trusted friend or relative will remember events you might have forgotten, will understand and remember treatment suggestions if you are very ill or confused, and will support you if the news is bad.

This is the single, most important portion of your examination, and you or your companion must explain concisely what is wrong with you. I stress the word "concisely," which means "no more than one sentence per complaint." If you ramble, are confused, or are unnecessarily wordy, your doctor may cut short your monologue. If he does, he could miss important information he needs to diagnose your problem.

He will ask you for specific details of your illness, but to his first question, "Why have you come to my office today?" you should say, "Because I suffer from headaches," if that is the case. Write down your symptoms and complaints before entering his office so you don't forget them. If you have other *main* reasons, then add them now. For example you might say, "I have headaches and blurry vision." Do not tell him your "neighbor down the block had a friend whose mother had a similar problem, and she...." Except in rare cases, he is not interested in your neighbor's illness and neither should you be.

Don't worry if you speak English poorly, your doctor will not (should not) ridicule the way you describe your symptoms. Experienced doctors have heard your problem explained in many ways, and many communicate in local dialects out of need. If you pass gas, say you pass gas, and not that your "microcosm is surrounded by pungent smells." He may think you are a fugitive from an oriental religious cult.

Neither should you disguise your private feelings, especially if they are the reason for your visit. If your sex-life is a disaster because you have pain on intercourse, do not say you always get a headache when your partner wants to have sex. If your pain is due to an ovarian tumor and your doctor orders a brain scan, you will delay therapy for a fatal illness. If you do not tell your doctor where to look, he will never uncover your problem much less correct it.

You may not know the medical name of your disease, but *you do know exactly what is wrong with you*. It is your doctor's responsibility to give a name to your disease, but it is your responsibility, and yours alone, to give him the information he needs to make that diagnosis.

Your Present Illness

This is where you describe your problem in detail. Since you need a well-planned presentation, you should record your symptoms carefully before entering his office. There is no set way to describe your illness, but your doctor will want to know when it started, the sequence of its symptoms, and its progression. About the last item, no matter how serious your symptoms were at first, if they are slowly disappearing, the odds are that your illness is not serious. Even if it is, be optimistic. You are on the road to recovery.

40

Your doctor will want to know how long you have been ill. An exact date is the most helpful, but unfortunately it is often not remembered in the case of slowly progressive diseases. If this is your situation, associate its onset to some event, such as the Christmas holidays, the notice of a penalty you owe on income taxes you forgot to pay, or a school graduation. By placing the beginning of your illness before or after such dates, you are still being helpful.

An example of a simple but complete answer to, "Why have you come to my office today?" may be: "About a month ago I started having headaches which would not go away with aspirin. Since then they have become more frequent and severe, and about ten days ago I started having blurred vision."

Precision and brevity are invaluable, and almost guarantee your doctor will diagnose your illness quickly and correctly.

He may interrupt you several times during the history as he explores different paths into the forest of your illness. There may be many causes for your symptoms, and not all of them will be life threatening. He may even ask the same questions several times. This is not because he is suffering from Alzheimer's disease, but because patients often immediately answer, "I do not remember." After a few minutes the question bumps into a fact they had forgotten, but by then they do not know how to present the newly remembered information without seeming foolish. His repetition of the question gives you the opportunity to look brilliant without embarrassment. ("It was a tough exam, but I answered all the questions," you will proudly tell your friends later.)

Now is also the time to present your fear of having cancer, AIDS, or whatever the panic disease of the month

41

is, as seen on TV. He may be able to tell you immediately if you have the disease you are worried about. Knowing you do not have cancer will make the rest of your interview go much more smoothly.

You may also *briefly* offer your solution to your problem. If one of your pupils is larger than the other and you think the cause might be your grandmother's eye drops you have been using, tell him. If your doctor does not ask if you are using eye drops, you may be hospitalized to treat a diabetic infarct of the third cranial nerve, even if you do not have diabetes.

At this point, you might want to ask your doctor about the medication you just read about in a full-page advertisement in *Star Magazine*, or whatever your source for medical information is. *Don't*. I will not prescribe drugs that are advertised for reasons I will explain in a later chapter, but for now, just know that most publicity sponsored by drug companies is underhanded and misleading, and is banned in the rest of the world. If your doctor thinks a new drug is useful, he'll prescribe it for you without your asking. If it *is* a wonder drug, I can assure you, he won't need you to tell him it exists. I often compare the patient who whines for a new drug to that of a spoiled kid in a toy shop, and I treat him so. Your doctor should prescribe medication *he* thinks you need, not what *you* think you need.

When a drug company resorts to direct consumer advertising, I stop prescribing its products in protest. It is easy to substitute one drug company's product with that of another, since many companies produce the same product under different trade names when patents expire. My patients will never suffer because of that substitution, and more importantly, will never become victims of new, unproven, and very costly drugs.

If you have already gone to a doctor who could not

solve your problem, have him forward your records to your new doctor. This will avoid unnecessary laboratory duplication and expense, and may save time, since it is likely that one or more of the possible causes of your disease already will have been eliminated. Your doctor may also use these records to monitor the course of your disease, since if an earlier test result is abnormally high, repeating it may show you are improving.

You should also know the names of *all* the medications you take on a daily, frequent, or occasional basis. This is much more important than you may think, as can be noted from the eye drop case. As a second example, you may have presumed that the fictional patient with headaches and blurry vision mentioned earlier in this chapter has a brain tumor. That is a possibility, but if this is your problem and you do not tell your doctor that you are a mega-vitamin freak, he will overlook the possibility of vitamin A toxicity as a cause.

In my practice, even though I specifically ask my patient what medications takes, he usually says "none." I leave a large space in my notes after that response, because I will add information to it later. Aspirin, birth control pills, vitamins, antacids, laxatives, and the myriad nonprescription products people consume daily are all medications and can cause an infinite number of problems. According to some statistics, bizarre reactions to medication are responsible for up to 20% of all hospitalizations.

If you remember all the drugs you take, you may avoid an expensive and unpleasant vacation in your local hospital. If you cannot remember their names, bring the bottles with you to your doctor's office.

Your Family History

Many diseases are handed down, like blue eyes, from mother to son. Some may skip a generation or two before reappearing, and knowing as much as you can about your family history will help. Your doctor will ask about your brothers and sisters, your parents, and your grandparents.

He will want to know about their health, if they are living or the cause of their deaths, and if there are any recurrent diseases in the family, such as cancer, heart disease, tuberculosis or diabetes. You should carefully research your family's general health history before your visit. If you have a fever, chronic cough, and weight loss, and forget your grandmother died last year of the same problem, you may undergo a work-up for lung cancer instead of tuberculosis.

Your Past Medical History

This section serves to bring your doctor up to date about your general health. He will ask about your past illnesses, vaccinations, infectious diseases, allergic reactions (chiefly to medications), hospitalizations and operations. The question about allergic reactions to medications is especially important, but too many of my patients know they are allergic to strawberries but do not know the name of a drug that made them seriously ill. Sadly, they do not even know why they took it.

One patient told me he was allergic to penicillin because he fainted after receiving an injection. In his case, he fainted was because he was allergic to the needle and not the antibiotic. Not all drug reactions are allergic in nature, and you should avoid condemning a valid medication. This is important if you need a drug your doctor will not prescribe because of your vague reaction to it.

Remember the name of any medication that has caused

you a problem in the past, since taking it again could be fatal. If you have trouble remembering, write down the name of the drug, the way you took it, and your exact reaction to it. Keep this information in your wallet so it will be handy should you ever need it.

Your Personal History

This consists of three parts: the first is your place of birth, home, and visits to foreign lands. If you think you picked up your rash on safari in Africa, tell your doctor. He knows the most common disease is always the most common, and if you don't give him an exotic cause, he might think you ate strawberries or were rolling in the hay with your partner.

Valley fever is a common disease in southern California, and in northern California when the winds blow the fungal spores to San Francisco. It is uncommon in Maine. If you were in a dust storm in Bakersfield last summer, now is the time to tell your doctor. Don't worry about the time lapse since your vacation. Not all infectious diseases appear immediately after contagion.

Next,\ he will ask about your habits, mostly your bad ones. If you help old people cross the street, this is unimportant unless you keep getting hit by cars. You must explain your smoking habits, coffee, diet, exercise, and drug use. Even though it's important to be honest about how much alcohol you drink or pot you smoke, most patients deliberately underestimate their use. Doctors automatically double or triple whatever you tell them. Unless you tell yours you know of this custom and tell him the quantity you describe is 100% accurate, you should change either your habit or your answer.

The last question in this category is about your weight

and eating habits. If you need to sit on two chairs side by side to support your bulk, no one will ever believe you eat like a bird. Eating habits can point directly to the cause of your illness, such as the case of a flight attendant who chewed 60 sticks of sugar-free gum daily and suffered from bouts of diarrhea. The gum contained sorbitol, a sugar the body cannot digest. Since it isn't absorbed, it carries a lot of water with it on its way out, and this caused her diarrhea.

Your Social History

This section documents your daily life. It will include your marital status, your occupation, including work conditions, emotional and physical responses to your job, and your home environment. These are important questions; do not take them lightly. I once examined a young woman who had been suffering from headaches, nausea and vomiting for a week before coming to see me.

She didn't tell me, even under direct questioning, that she had remodeled her bedroom ten days earlier, and the chemicals she used to remove the old wallpaper in the room were the cause of her symptoms. They made her sick, and then kept her in bed to make sure she remained ill.

Your Review of Systems

This is the last portion of the interview. He will question you about each of your body's systems and your interpretation of the way they work. The questioning may vary, as a dermatologist may begin with your skin and a neurologist with your head, but from that point on it becomes routine. He will ask you specific questions about your chest, abdomen, circulation, and I hope your sex-life, if that is the purpose of your visit and you were too embarrassed to

46

bring it up before now.

This ends your colloquial, but before moving on to the physical section of your visit, your doctor will ask if you have questions, doubts, or comments. This is your last chance to tell your story; do not let the moment slip by because of fear, embarrassment, or intimidation. The life you save will be your own!

Now begins the hands on portion of the examination. There is no set program for this either, since each doctor will develop a favorite routine. The main goal, however, is to examine all of your anatomy in as much detail as possible without causing pain or damage. If you are still wearing your overcoat at this point, your doctor is not performing the examination correctly.

Specialists focus their examination on a single organ system, whereas a family practitioner's examination is general in scope. For example, a gynecologist will perform a pelvic and a Pap smear routinely but will not check your teeth; a family practitioner would do both, and a neurologist would do neither. Since a complete neurological examination can take more than an hour, you would hope a neurologist would not take the time to count your molars. If he did, a late morning appointment could ruin your afternoon television soap operas. This does not mean you are being slighted. If you have chosen a competent general practitioner, he should have performed a physical examination before referring you to a specialist.

After he has recorded and evaluated your history and physical, your doctor should have a good idea about your illness. At this point he may order laboratory examinations to confirm his diagnosis. Accept his suggestion to immediate testing *only* if your disease is an emergency or requires urgent intervention. If it is not so dramatic, I would suggest you first follow my recommendations in the chapters "How to Cure Your Doctor" and "It's Your Health Dollar."

For those of you who would like to know the history of some of the gadgets your doctor will want to use on you if you cannot come up with a delaying tactic, the following is a brief tour of the endless array of more or less sophisticated instruments which will bump, grind, and glow their way to the diagnosis and treatment of your disease:

We owe the discovery of the stethoscope to R. T. H. Laennec. In 1816 he wrote about the difficulties he encountered while examining a young lady with heart disease:

> In her case the application of the hand was out of the question because of a considerable degree of stoutness (a gentile way of describing her obesity). Listening to the sounds within the chest by the direct application of the ear to the chest wall was inadmissible by the age and sex of the patient.
>
> I rolled a quire of paper into a cylinder and applied one end of it to the region of the heart and the other to my ear. I was not a little surprised and pleased to find that I could hear the action of the heart in a manner much more clear and distinct than I had ever been able to do by the immediate application of the ear.

After the demand for quires fell into decline, a wooden cylinder replaced it, and the stethoscope, or the ears of medicine, was born. Dr. Laennec's invention is the most commonly used instrument in medicine today.

All medical instruments, as all therapies, have both intended uses and unexpected or unwanted results. The stethoscope enables the doctor to hear sounds produced by the body's organs he cannot hear with his naked ear alone, or the violation of decorum described by Dr. Laennec would prevent him from hearing. Its unintended function is that it may be a germ carrier without equal.

A problem I noted with alarming regularity is that of the elderly patient who boasts that he has not been ill with the flu since Roosevelt was president. For some reason he feels guilty about not having had a checkup in thirty years and comes into my office for a routine physical. With a precision you could set your watch by, he calls three days after his visit to tell me he is ill, and asks me to prescribe something for his symptoms. While I cannot be sure the stethoscope I used to listen to his heart was the cause, doubtless he got his disease in my office.

Another common instrument is the electrocardiograph, or ECG. This machine's primary use is to determine the nature of certain forms of heart disease, although I have seen a colleague order it on a patient with low back pain. He could not explain its exact role in his diagnosis of this problem.

We will never know the percentage of wrong diagnoses created or of true diagnoses missed by this machine, but a guess of 25% in either direction would not be an exaggeration. The implication is enormous and can have a lasting effect on your psyche. How do you live a normal life if an EKG tells you your healthy heart is sick, or your sick heart is healthy?

There are many other "standardizers" in your doctor's office. These serve to collect data whose primary function is to tell (and alarm) you that you deviate from the average human being by a precise number of inches, pounds, or millimeters of mercury. I am not sure why people prefer being identical members of a herd rather than individuals, but it is not uncommon for an infant who weighs a pound or two less than his average peer to be forced to drink extra bottles of expensive formula until he catches up to him.

The child will gain weight, but the obese creature that now corresponds exactly to the weight tables no longer resembles the trim figure it once was.

After you complete your history, physical, and tour through the laboratory, your doctor will tell you the name of your disease and his proposed cure. This is an important moment. Under the legal doctrine of informed consent, he must tell you the risks, benefits, and alternatives to the treatment he suggests in a language you understand.

Presuming he does, what do you do with his advice, for which you may have just paid a month's salary and may be incorrect? You evaluate it, of course, just as you would any other important piece of information. I'll tell you how to do this later, but statistics show you will either not follow his advice, or you will do so until you feel better and then quit. Statistics are often unreliable but these are important since others do not show that one in two patients dies because he does not follow his doctor's instructions to the letter.

This proves that doctors and their therapies are not always correct. However, relapses of ulcers, rashes, and infections can occur if you stop taking your medication sooner than you should. You may try to shirk the blame if your disease returns, but if your doctor's diagnosis and therapy were correct and you changed his therapy to suit yourself, the fault of his treatment failure is yours alone.

To avoid either a relapse or severe complications, and at the same time to decide how much treatment you do need, you must understand your illness. Your doctor must explain your disease in detail, why he feels his therapy is necessary, and what he reasonably expects will occur if you do not follow his instructions precisely.

If he explains this to you in Medicalese, have him translate it into English.

Chapter Four

"There are...more old drunkards than old
physicians."
Rabelais: Gargantua I.xli.

Life is full of health problems that most often include
tiredness, headache, low back pain, gas, arthritis, and con-
stipation. You can extract these thorns by simple cures that
do not include drilling holes in your skull, as primitive doctors did to relieve the demon spirits they believed were
causing their patients' headaches.

Some doctors distinguish minor from major symptoms
better than others. Specialists are experts in their fields, but
know little about diseases are outside their fields. In fact
they are the least qualified to diagnose and treat the vast
number of problems that besiege our everyday lives, yet
their number grows while the general practitioner, the bul-
wark of the profession, goes the way of the Edsel.

Specialists are not infallible, but because they know a
lot about a little, their diagnosis of your problem is often
accepted without question. This can be to your detriment,
as reported in the study of a group of impotent men. Psy-
chiatrists found an emotional basis for their impotency,

urologists a mechanical cause, and endocrinologists a glandular cause. Drug companies now presume that all men over thirty are impotent and have invented their own disease and given it a very fancy name: erectile dysfunction. They have even invented an expensive medication to "cure" it.

That's four different diagnoses and four different therapies for the same problem in the same patients. As was recounted in *Tom Jones*, each doctor has his favorite disease. An interesting idea, but not when *your* sex life is at stake.

Another example is Eileen who arrived in my emergency room complaining of pain in her left arm. Since she was under the care of a cardiologist for this problem, my nurse put her in the coronary care room and put her on a heart monitor. Besides her alleged heart disease, she told me an orthopedic surgeon was treating her left leg problem that had been worsening over a period of months.

After my examination, I realized a growth on the right side of her brain would explain both her arm and leg problems and that she did not have heart disease. A brain scan revealed a 3/4-inch diameter tumor that was successfully removed at surgery.

Her specialists missed her diagnosis because they had been treating her as if she were made of dissociated organs. This is an ineffective and expensive way to practice medicine, and could have resulted in her premature death.

Since most of your illnesses will resolve on their own, it is statistically unimportant whether specialists agree on your diagnosis or not. What is important is that their different diagnostic tools can put your life at risk. The cardiologist, eager to run a catheter into your heart because you're male and belched after age 40, is not doing you a favor.

Let's trail behind a 45 year-old patient with a healthy heart who visits a marginally competent cardiologist because of chest pain. Most of us know that a burning sensation behind the breastbone will disappear rapidly after taking an antacid. However, there are those who will run to the doctor for this symptom before taking any medication, even those sold over-the-counter. Their heartburn needs in-office treatment.

Even though our fictitious patient's ECG will not reveal heart disease, if he is insured his cardiologist will convince him to undergo a dangerous test "just to be sure" his heart is healthy. A coronary angiogram (or arteriogram) is an X-ray of the heart's arteries taken after a catheter injects dye into them. The indications for this procedure are listed in any medical textbook, as I will explain later in detail.

After his angiogram, his cardiologist will warn him he may suffer a heart attack if he does not have surgery for the minor defects he will always find on the X-ray. In the sad case of a friend of mine, his doctor couldn't find any defects on his angiogram, so he invented them, convincing him to undergo surgery twice for his symptoms. Neither relieved his pain; quitting his stressful job did.

The surgeries for clogged heart arteries include coronary bypass surgery and coronary angioplasty. The former replaces the blocked artery with a graft, often a vein taken from your legs or your chest. Candidates for this procedure must have both a heart and an insurance policy.

A limiting factor in the number of these operations is that the surgeon must open the patient's chest to get to his heart. The thought of a large scar running zipper-like down the middle of their chest is enough to deter many patients from undergoing the operation.

To overcome this obstacle, medical cardiologists invented coronary angioplasty, a simplified version of the bypass operation. Patients must have the same qualifications as those needed for bypass surgery, but in this case, they insert a catheter into the patient's leg or wrist artery and then feed it into the arteries around his heart. When it bumps into a cholesterol plaque, they inflate a balloon at its tip, crushing it against the walls of the artery.

Since they occasionally rupture the artery during the procedure, a cardiovascular surgeon stands by, ready to perform the "zipper" operation if this calamity occurs. This doubles the patient's anxiety and his medical bill. Six months after this procedure, the artery will return to its prior clogged state in a high percentage of cases unless weight reduction, diet change, exercise, and the elimination of bad habits, especially smoking, accompany the procedure. These are the real cures for the problem.

In this example, since we know the patient had heartburn, which has nothing to do with the heart, the cardiologist's diagnosis was wrong and his unnecessary treatment could have had tragic results. If the situation does not sound appealing, it could have been even worse if *you* were the patient and your problem was indigestion.

To arrive at a solution to any health problem, major or minor, you must first find a qualified general practitioner or his counterpart, the family practitioner, as described in chapter two. He may not be able to quote obscure articles in cardiology journals, but he will be able to tell you if your problem is your heart, your stomach, or your mind. He will also know when to refer you to a specialist. Last, but not least importantly, if your disease is incurable, he, above all others, can console you.

The difficulty comes after your doctor completes your history and physical examinations and suggests a diagnosis. Now, you must decide if he is correct. It's obvious that if he isn't, the tests he orders and the therapy he proposes will be wrong also.

Surgery is the correct treatment for appendicitis but not

for indigestion. Therefore, before accepting your doctor's diagnosis, you must verify that it and his proposed laboratory tests and treatment plan are all correct. The market is awash with books to help you diagnose your disease. In some you just look up your symptom in the index and read the diagnosis.

Unfortunately, even the most basic books fall short of their goal because you lack the experience necessary to interpret and to catalog your symptoms correctly. Yet, once you have the name of your disease, it will be easy to refer to them or to the Internet, to see if its symptoms match yours. There you will also learn about its causes, diagnostic requirements, treatment, and outcome.

Detailed but limited in scope volumes, such as Lange's *Current Medical Diagnosis & Treatment*, the *Physicians' Desk Reference* (the PDR), and many others, will help. Lange's is a medical textbook written in Medicalese, but it is an excellent means to confirm your doctor's diagnosis and his proposed treatment. Do not feel guilty about not understanding Medicalese; it is a language invented to humble the layperson. If Lange's book is too sophisticated for you, search for one written in a style you are more comfortable with, such as family medical encyclopedia.

Many of the diseases described in these texts have unhappy endings, as does life itself; ignore them. People who are dying know they are, and have no need to read about their illnesses. Being concerned means you are still in satisfactory health and will work in your favor.

I am not suggesting you use these books to arrive at a diagnosis on your own. It will be almost impossible for you to use specialized texts efficiently until *after* you know your diagnosis. This is the same for a beginner in any field, from aardvark anatomy to zymurgical aberrations.

Rather I am suggesting you use them to confirm your

diagnosis, and your doctor's request for a test or treatment that seems extreme or unusual for your symptoms or your pocketbook. If you want to try to diagnose your disease, you will need a simpler, cookbook style textbook that describes a symptom followed by a flow sheet.

This may not help you arrive at a diagnosis either, but Vickery and Fields', *Take Care of Yourself, A Consumer's Guide to Medical Care*, tells you when to seek immediate aid and when to apply home treatment. If you can treat yourself, great! But if you do need help, then Vickery and Fields' book goes on the back shelf and the others take its place.

If you're adventurous you might try to diagnose your problem with a medical test you can buy in a drugstore. This could be a happy experience if you want to know if you're pregnant, but it could be disastrous if you're testing yourself for AIDS. If you intend to become a home chemist, you should remember a few basic principles:

1. Carefully read and understand the directions on the container. Don't skip any steps you think are unnecessary.

2. Follow any special precautions the manufacturer recommends, such as avoiding certain foods or medicines before the testing.

3. Check the expiration date. There is usually a little leeway between the actual expiration date and the date on the box, but why take chances? Do not use out-of-date reagents since they can give both false positive and false negative results, meaning you don't have what they say you do, or do have what they say you don't. Confusing? Think of the effect either result will have on your life if you think you're pregnant and don't want to be. If in doubt, repeat the test with fresh reagents.

4. If a local supermarket has a two for one sale on pregnancy tests and you don't intend to use both of them

the same day, make sure to properly store the one you don't use. If it needs to be refrigerated, don't leave it in the trunk of your car.

5. If you notice a white powder on your food during your divorce and decide to test the arsenic content of your hair, remember that precision is essential. If the directions require a stopwatch, make sure you have one. I knew of a laboratory that used a stopwatch without hands to time the tests it ran. Accuracy in that laboratory was abysmal, but then the technicians weren't testing the blood of their loved ones. I'll talk more about this later, but for now, remember that precision counts.

6. Decide beforehand if you want to be alone or in the company of friends to share the news when the test results are in.

7. Before you let bad results get you down, talk with your doctor or pharmacist, or call the company that makes the product for advice. You may have performed it incorrectly or are doing something that will give false results. If you think you'll need to call the company, perform the test during its working hours. In any case, repeat the test before drawing up your last Will and Testament.

Accompanying you to the doctor with imaginary chest pain, I will show you how you can use the information I presented so far to your advantage, and how to avoid the travails of the uninformed patient with heartburn I described earlier.

Let us presume you are male, fifty years old, have just finished lunch, and are walking back to your office. A few minutes after you begin your fast pace down Main Street, you are gripped by severe pain behind your breastbone. You sit on a bench along the curb, cursing yourself for not kissing your spouse good-by that morning. The pain passes in a few minutes and you resume your walk, but it returns a short time later.

You're fairly sure your heart is the cause of your pain, but since it passes again and does not return, when you get home you hug your wife tightly, tell her you love her and apologize for all the bad things you've ever done to her before pulling Dr. Vickery's book off the shelf. Based on your symptoms, he tells you your pain may be significant and he suggests you see your doctor immediately. This is good advice and you should follow it.

Let's also presume that during your first meeting with a new family doctor, he questions and examines you, and performs an ECG that would have confirmed the diagnosis of angina pectoris (heart pain) had you had the pain during the test. Since you were pain free at the time, your ECG was normal.

Your doctor will order blood tests, including cardiac enzymes, cholesterol and sugar levels, and may even agree to order the tests described in last week's *Woman's Day Magazine* if you press him hard enough. The fly on the wall in his office has too often heard his patients ask, "Do you think it's my polystyrene, Doc? Should I add raw oatmeal to my bacon chip and sour cream salads? How about that new medicine I saw advertised on TV last night for chest pain and erectile dysfunction? Will you write me a prescription?"

You, savvy as you are, will not request any of the above. After an explanation of your probable disease and a review of your laboratory tests, your doctor will refer you to a cardiologist with the presumed diagnosis of angina pectoris. Ask him to write down the medical name of your suspected disease (printing it may make its translation easier). Since you are pain free, before going to the cardiologist and undergoing any dangerous or expensive tests, and after you immediately stop smoking, your next step is to find out if his diagnosis of angina pectoris is correct. This is not difficult, and you can quickly corroborate or exclude it.

Lange describes the symptoms of "Angina Pectoris" as: "...squeezing or pressure-like pain, retrosternal or slightly to the left, that appears quickly during exertion, may radiate in a set pattern, and subsides with rest."

This means the cramp-like pain starts behind your breastbone, appears quickly while you are physically active, may travel in the same direction each time it appears (for example, to your jaw or down your left arm), and disappears quickly at rest.

If you had difficulty understanding this description in Lange, search for a simpler text. If you had no trouble with it, learn a few Latin phrases, and you can pass for one of us at some dull party.

Do your symptoms agree with those described in the text? If they do, your disease is angina pectoris and you should visit the specialist. If they have nothing in common with Lange's description, consult a different general practitioner.

In your case, you have angina pectoris, and your stress test (an ECG performed while you walk a treadmill), will confirm this. Your first ECG was normal because you were pain free when you had it performed.

Now that we have correctly diagnosed your illness, the next step is treatment. You will want only that which is necessary and in your best interests. In general, if the therapy your doctor proposes seems reasonable, inexpensive, and safe, you can start it immediately. If it seems drastic, inappropriate, or expensive and there is no emergency, postpone it until you can evaluate it. (A helpful hint: expensive therapies and treatments are more often unnecessary than are inexpensive prescriptions.)

Let's suppose your cardiologist recommends immediate coronary angiography. How do you know if you need it or not? Lange states its "most common indication is unacceptable angina pectoris unimproved by restricted activity, nitrates, beta-blocking, or calcium entry-blocking agents."

Therefore, you need to undergo a trial of medication before agreeing to angiography. This is a necessity! You may not know what those medications are (you will before you finish this book), but Lange is telling you that angiography is not for you. Even later, if your symptoms are mild in that you can walk, exercise, or have no limits to your normal activities while taking medication, you still will not need the angiogram and you should not have it performed.

An angiogram is not therapy, has never saved a life, and carries a 0.1% mortality and a 1-5% morbidity risk by provoking the heart attack you are trying to prevent. A rule to remember about angiograms, myelograms or any other potentially dangerous, invasive procedures (where something is injected or inserted into your body) is that they are used to determine if you would benefit from surgery if your disease were not adequately controlled by other means. If you intend to refuse surgery or other therapy, no matter what the results of the procedure, there is no point in having it done. Undergoing an expensive and dangerous test just to complete your work-up is not worth the possibility of injury or death.

Also, there is an undesirable result of this testing. If you did have a bout of indigestion, you may become a psychological cardiac cripple (cardiac neurosis) if your doctor warns you that your heart might be diseased even without abnormal findings.

If an unethical cardiologist has persuaded you to undergo the angiogram before documenting your response to medication, he may also try to convince you that you could suffer a heart attack if you do not have surgery for the defect he allegedly found on the X-ray. How do you know if you need it? Lange states of coronary angioplasty, "as with coronary bypass surgery, patients should have disabling angina pectoris not responding adequately to medical treatment." Therefore, if your disease is not disabling, you do not need the procedure. Even if it is disabling, before consenting to surgery you must still reduce your weight, quit smoking (coronary surgery is not a cure for the nicotine habit), and take your medication.

The suggestion to have surgery will be subtle of course, since protocol requires you undergo a trial of medication before running the risks of a possibly fatal procedure. Subtle or not, if your cardiologist's advice goes against that described in a reliable textbook of medicine, go to another, the best your budget allows, since the cost of a consultation by an honest individual will be far less than the proposed surgery.

Suppose your doctor has followed all the current theories about treating your angina, and has prescribed Procardia, a well-known and respected medication used in to treat this disease. After several weeks of therapy your pain has disappeared and you are back playing touch football, but because your legs are swollen up to your knees, your doctor now wants to hospitalize you to perform a venogram. This is an X-ray of your legs after dye is injected into the veins of your feet to find out if there is a blockage in your leg veins. Do you agree? Of course not! As you will learn in a later chapter, you must presume any symptoms that develop after you start taking a new medication are due to that medication until proven otherwise.

Ask your doctor to write down the name of your new symptom. In this case it is peripheral edema. This is where you need your PDR (*Physicians' Desk Reference*), or more commonly the Internet. Look up the name of your medication, Procardia, in the pink pages of the PDR or online, and then search for "precautions," or "adverse reactions." The information you seek is under precautions. Under the subheading "Peripheral Edema" it states, "mild to moderate peripheral edema...occurs in about one in ten patients treated with Procardia." This is your problem. Stop the medicine and your peripheral edema will disappear in a few days. If it does not, then search for other reasons for it.

Angina is not the most common problem you will face in your life, but external hemorrhoids are. Like most of your ailments, these will disappear in seven days with therapy or in a week without, and your doctor's treatment is unimportant. Unless it is wrong. By referring to the texts, you'll learn that his prescription for antibiotics to treat them is inappropriate (and absurd).

Avoiding unnecessary therapy is an important step in preserving your physical and financial health. But if you constantly have to correct your doctor's diagnoses and therapies for minor problems, you will not want him treating your more serious ones, especially in an emergency. You will feel uncomfortable when you are semi-comatose, hear him offer his opinion at your bedside, and know you cannot move your shattered body to your library or desktop computer to corroborate his diagnosis and therapy.

One final point: competent doctors do err in diagnosis and treatment. However, they differ from their lesser-qualified brethren because their mistakes are few, rapidly corrected, and are easily explainable when the facts are brought to light. Therefore, before criticizing your doctor, remember diseases can worsen over time and diagnosis by hindsight is easy. Unfortunately, his daily decisions are not. His greatest frustration is that he cannot control destiny.

The flu is a common, seasonal malady. It is an annoying break in your daily schedule, but most people overcome it in a few days. Unfortunately, for a few, a simple cough and fever today can worsen into bronchopneumonia tomorrow, pericarditis (an infection of the lining around the heart) the day after, and death by the end of the week.

On the first day of this common viral illness, a competent practitioner might suggest medications such as aspirin, cough syrup, and fluids for the relief of your symptoms. On the second day he would prescribe an antibiotic to cure the bronchopneumonia. Had you called him on the third day, your problem would be more complex, but with proper care you would survive. Had you waited until the end of the week to call for help, well, sorry, you waited too long.

Now let's suppose that instead of calling the same doctor each day, you call a different one. The first two will suggest the same remedies mentioned above; the third will exclaim, "Pericarditis!" and demand immediate hospitalization. The fourth will fill in the forms needed in cases of unexpected death.

Each correctly arrived at a different diagnosis and prescribed a correct treatment for the disease at the moment he saw you. Where they differ is in their professional behavior. Let's suppose, Dr. Brown, doctor number three, does not tell you pericarditis may complicate the flu and that taking antibiotics routinely cannot prevent it and may be dangerous. In fact he tells you none of the above, but he does tell you his first two colleagues erred in their diagnosis and treatment, and that he is the best doctor in the entire state.

The result is that while you are dialing your lawyer, you keep repeating to yourself that the first and second doctors were wrong, and "Thank God for Dr. Brown!"

Could the first doctors have treated you better? Should doctor number one have prescribed unnecessary antibiotics, simply to place himself in a legally defensible position? Should he have hospitalized you and ordered a battery of tests to convince you his diagnosis was correct? Or to convince your heirs and their lawyers that he had examined every possibility in your care? Should he have warned you that you might develop pericarditis, needlessly increasing your concern about your illness? Should have signed the death certificate and have left it by your bedside?

This "simple" illness shows that a doctor's life is not easy, and that criticism of his care in hindsight may be unjust. The flu is unresponsive to modern therapy and will resolve on its own, although age, prior health, physical condition, and domestic surroundings can alter its generally benign outcome. Its treatment in the early stages is based on the doctor's art and not his scientific knowledge. The cures he proposes before complications set in are no more effective than Grandma's chicken soup and her innumerable trips to the bedside to fluff your pillow and to make sure the wet rag on your forehead is still cool. (As a point of interest, grandmothers and mothers understand instinctively any change in a family member's health before it becomes obvious to anybody else. They should never allow the seeming superiority of experts to suppress their instincts.)

Medicine is not an exact science. Although the wiles of the unethical, and the voids of the incompetent practitioner are fathomless, you can still turn the odds of survival in your favor by choosing your doctor carefully, and by being thoroughly informed about your illness and its proposed therapy.

As in all else, in medicine you get what you pay for. Do not let the price include life or limb.

Chapter Five

TAKE YOUR MEDICINE:
Deciding on the Right Medications

"Some remedies are worse than the disease."
Publilius Syrus: Maxims.

A mother once asked me how to lower her child's fever. I explained to her what my mother did to lower mine when I was young, and I asked her to call me back if it didn't work or if her child developed other symptoms.

Several days later, I ran into her on the street and asked how her child was, and if she had followed my suggestions. She answered sheepishly, "Well, no. I rubbed an egg all over my baby's body. When it was cooked, her fever was gone."

So much for modern medicine! However, it proved a point. Ignoring their frequent side effects and sometimes outrageous costs, most medications prescribed to treat minor illnesses are unnecessary.

The use of drugs to cure disease is not a new idea. In ancient Egypt physician priests were divided into two classes: one made house calls and the other prepared remedies in the temple. The same arrangement exists today, except few modern doctor priests make house calls.

In Bruges in 1683 the law forbade doctors to dispense

prescriptions. Today's doctor can if he wishes, but he usually has a pharmacist do it for him. Some, however, sell medications to their patients, thus protesting the pharmacist's tendency to assume the role of doctor when his client seeks medical advice. Some doctors protest so loudly that they sell the clearly marked "not for sale" free samples drug sales representatives give to them.

Years ago, I knew a pharmacist who was guilty of the same crime, although why a pharmaceutical house had given him free samples eludes me, since he only could fill prescriptions, not write them.

Not long ago a drug representative was convicted of a scheme to sell samples at cut-rate prices to seven pharmacists from Connecticut. All eight of them were fined and had their licenses suspended or revoked. Some served sentences of home confinement. This was in addition to five others who had previously been convicted in the same case.

Consumers were defrauded because the sample drugs sold lacked the labeling information required by law, including the expiration dates and lot numbers that were not transferred from the sample containers to the patient packages.

Until early in this century, most drugs, if not especially effective, were at least safe, although the pharmaceutical industry produced medications that most people today would consider distasteful, as Alexander H. Ross, M.D. wrote in his 1888 monograph, *Fallacies and Delusions of the Medical Profession:*

From another standard medical work, "Collecteanæ Medica," London, 1725, page 26, we find the following remedies: For Quinsy: powder of burnt owls, two drachms; burnt swallows, one drachm; cat's brains, two drachms; dried and powdered blood of white puppy dogs, two drachms. For Colic: wolf's guts dried and powdered, two drachms; old man's urine, three drachms; sheep's excrements, two drachms; a sovereign remedy.

We're beholden to the industry for its decision to cease butchering our pets and livestock in its historical quest to cure our ills, however, many of its modern synthetic substitutes, while palatable, are much more powerful, dangerous and deadly. The margin between dose and overdose has narrowed, and Shakespeare's phrase, "in poison there is physic" has renewed meaning. If you remember that *all* medicines are poisons that must enter and alter your body's cells if they are to do their job, and if you evaluate them carefully before you take them, you may avoid many of their unpleasant side effects and save money as well.

It is also worth remembering that often the difference between a medication and a poison is the simply its dosage.

While you may never need to take medication, if you should someday, remember the following principles:

1. Your body will survive most of its diseases *and* their therapies on its own, therefore taking nothing will cure you most of the time. If your doctor cannot or need not treat your problem, he should tell you this and not offer you useless therapy, such as an antibiotic to cure the flu. It is easier for your body to fight its disease alone than to fight its disease and a toxic drug.

Since many patients feel they cannot recover without taking "something" (or worse, think their "doctor don't know nottin', 'cause he don't give no pills."), many office visits end with a prescription. This misunderstanding of what you think your doctor should do for you is one of the prime causes of "iatrogenic disease." Webster defines this as "a disease, which is induced inadvertently to the patient by a physician or his treatment."

You pay your doctor *for his opinion and not for a prescription*. If he says you have disease "X" and you will recover in a few days without treatment, believe him.

To avoid unnecessary side effects, take medication

only if you need it to cure your illness. Do not ask for one if your doctor does not offer it. If he does, ask him why you need it, how to take it, and any side effects you might experience. If he adds you'll recover without it, ask him why he's prescribing it. Then watch him squirm as he tries to invent a reason to explain his decision to give you a drug you didn't need.

If you are a hypochondriac who fantasizes symptoms and know you will get every side effect your doctor describes, have him explain the potential problems to the friend or relative who accompanied you to his office. Then, if you think the pink pill is causing blue hair to grow rapidly up your chest, do not wait until it reaches your eyebrows. Tell your friend about it! If he agrees with you, or is not sure, check your PDR or the Internet, which I'll discuss later, for information on drug side effects.

If you can't find the answer there, call your doctor or your pharmacist and ask him if psychedelic hirsutism is a side effect of the drug. If he is unsure or unavailable, stop the medication until you get a satisfactory answer to your question.

As mentioned in an earlier chapter, *any symptoms you did not have before you started your medication are due solely to that medication until proven otherwise.* If the blue hair on your chest recedes when you stop your medication, proving it was a side effect, and if you really do need a drug to treat your illness, ask your doctor to prescribe something that will not make you to look like a kaleidoscopic gorilla. If there is no substitute, ask him if he will pay your barber bill. *Do not consent to undergo laboratory examinations, take another medication, or consent to hospitalization for a work-up, unless you are certain the medication did not cause the hairy growth.*

2. No drug, except possibly vitamin C, is free of side

effects. In fact, drugs often are prescribed to take advantage of them, such as diet pills. The over-the-counter brands have names reminiscent of the amphetamines doctors pre-scribed years ago, but are simple allergy pills that cause a decrease in appetite. At least you would hope that to be the case. *St. Joseph's Cold Tablets for Children* and *Dexatrim* weight control tablets are chemically identical, except the St. Joseph's tablet also contains aspirin. Side effects such as appetite suppression are minimal and at times may be wel-comed, but others can be severe or unpleasant. You must accept them if the drug is to perform its primary purpose. If you cannot, have your doctor change your medication.

One drug consumed in great quantities by a large per-centage of the population has the following side effects: one person in five-hundred will suffer a severe allergic re-action to it, such as angioneurotic edema (swelling of the face), hives, skin rash, a form of asthma that may be fatal, or rare true anaphylactic shock with collapse (similar to what happens after a bee sting). Gastrointestinal bleeding of one teaspoonful a day, if the drug is taken according to directions, occurs in 70% of those who use it. High doses cause nausea, stomach upset, vomiting, and ringing in the ears. Extended use of the drug may cause certain blood cells not to work properly, resulting in postoperative hem-orrhage, prolonged menstrual periods, and kidney or liver disease. At one time in England, 200 people a year used the drug to commit suicide.

Studies have suggested that children who take this medication during febrile illnesses such as chicken pox, risk developing Reye's syndrome, a tragic, but rare compli-cation of that disease.

Can you guess the name of this "killer" drug?

It is aspirin. Since this is considered to be a safe medi-cation, you can buy it anywhere.

3. Since all medications have side effects, some doctors prescribe other medications to counteract them before they occur, or as quickly as they occur. They are known as an "add-on doctors." Avoid them. Rather than evaluate the effects of their medications one at a time, they immediately prescribe several all at once. If his multiple medications do not produce the wanted results, rather than discontinue or substitute them, he simply adds another.

His treatment of hypertension is an example of his penchant to over treat. Potassium loss (hypokalemia) *may* occur following the long-term use of diuretics or "water pills." Even though it usually takes six to nine months for this to happen with the milder drugs, the add-on physician routinely prescribes potassium supplements when he prescribes a diuretic. He does this even knowing you can avoid hypokalemia by simply including high potassium foods in your diet, such as bananas, orange juice, and the skin of a baked potato. Thus you take two drugs instead of one, spending twice as much as you need to, and doubling your risk of side effects. To make matters worse, too much potassium will stop your heart dead in its tracks, literally. It's one of the drugs some states use to execute criminals "humanely."

The most extravagant example of this is the patient who took *15* medications a day. Needing only two to treat his illness, his doctor told me he prescribed the other 13 to correct the side effects of those two pills and some of his add on medications *before* they occurred. Another rule is that unless you are extremely ill, and even if you are, most prescriptions over two are unnecessary.

You can reach your goal of taking the least amount of medicine necessary to treat your illness by finding a "substitute-pill" doctor, one who will begin your therapy with a low potency medication that has been around for many years. If he does not get the results he wants, he will stop his first medication before prescribing the next one up the ladder of cost and peril. He may "add-on" medication, but only rarely, for specific reasons, and never simply to anticipate a side effect that you might never even develop.

Medications prescribed to cure the potential or real side effects of other medications is an eternal, dangerous, and expensive game. Almost 20% of all hospitalizations are due to drug reactions, and the "diseases" they cause can be difficult and costly to diagnose, since the symptoms and signs they produce do not fit the descriptions of textbook illnesses. Stopping them before running "all the tests just to be sure," will usually resolve the iatrogenic disease immediately.

If you feel your doctor is over-prescribing, confront him. If he insists you take all his medications simply because one pill corrects the side effects of the other, seek a second opinion before you get into trouble.

4. If you need to take a medication, ask your doctor if the one he is prescribing is an old standby with many years of proven effectiveness and safety behind it, or if it is a new drug a pharmaceutical representative has just dropped off in his office. Drug representatives constantly badger doctors with their newest products, insisting what they peddle is much better than their competitors' and their side effects are less serious or nonexistent.

There will always be a new product to sell tomorrow, and despite its glitter, the odds overwhelmingly favor that by the time the last doctor in town learns of the new wonder drug, a next generation, more potent, and more dangerous one will have replaced it. And since drug companies have to recover the costs of the promotional perks they give doctors to help them remember their drug's name before its demise, it is invariably expensive. Although it is now theoretically illegal, these perks include(d) Caribbean cruises, multi-thousand dollar computer systems, and $200.00 a plate dinners. I know of one doctor who prescribes so much medication that drug salesmen buy lunch for him and his staff every day of the week. They recover the costs of these meals if he prescribes their medications only twice a month.

Some doctors prescribe new medications without the slightest idea of their cost, side effects, and contraindications. Drug representatives never volunteer this information, and doctors rarely take the time to read the warnings and incomplete list of contraindications printed on the medication's information sheet.

Often a specialist is the first to prescribe a new drug for his patients whose diseases have not responded to older medications. It is often the only tool he has to separate him from a competent family practitioner.

An example of is Oraflex, an arthritis medication alleged to have contributed to the deaths of over 100 people during the first year of its release in the United States decades ago. The drug company alleged that doctors themselves caused those deaths by prescribing the drug in large doses to patients who should not have received it at all. Even if this was so, this drug and the entire group of antiarthritic drugs, known as NSAID or nonsteroidal anti-inflammatory drugs, have never been proven to be more effective than plain aspirin in relieving arthritis pains, even though their side effects are the same. I have already explained what aspirin can do to you.

As to pricing, the cost of generic aspirin is pennies a day. One company's expensive brand of aspirin allegedly may enter the bloodstream faster than its competitor's, but that does not guarantee it will work faster. Even if it did, the few seconds' advantage is hardly worth the difference in cost.

The average price of prescription antiarthritic medications on the other hand, is $1.00 a day if taken according to recommended dosages. The drug industry has standardized that cost: if you need to take it once a day, it will cost $1.00 a pill. Do you need two? The cost drops to 50 cents a pill. Three pills a day? Then each pill costs 34 cents. This is known as friendly competition.

Another interesting idea is marketing prescription drugs for over-the-counter sales (OTC). Ibuprofen, the chemical name of the active ingredient of Motrin, Advil, Genpril, Ibu-200, Midol, and Nuprin among others, is an anti-inflammatory drug commonly used to treat fevers and minor arthritic pains, although it has recently fallen into disrepute because of a newly discovered side effect: it can cause a heart attack and kill you.

You can buy it over-the-counter, in 200 mg. doses. To get the 400 mg. or 800 mg. pills, you need a prescription. Most patients can figure out that two 200 mg. pills equals one 400 mg. pill, and that four 200 mg. pills equals one 800 mg. pill, so there must be another reason for needing a prescription.

Doubling or tripling the OTC pills will cost less than the prescription and will save you a doctor's bill. A word of caution, however: long-term use of this drug in high doses will destroy your kidneys. Also, the 800 mg. tablet is no more effective than are the 400 mg. or 600 mg. tablets. The higher dosage will not give you greater pain relief, only greater complications.

The use of a "new" medication in its most Machiavellian guise is when a doctor tells you "a new drug to help your disease will be on the market in a month. To get it as soon as possible, schedule an appointment with the receptionist on your way out."

This scheme has a dual effect: it keeps your hopes up that a cure for your chronic health problem is near, and it keeps his waiting room filled. He can keep his promise because new drugs do appear on the market regularly, and when patents run out on the old ones, competing companies produce them under different names.

Unless you are astute enough to know the chemical names of the medicines you take, an unscrupulous practitioner will fool you every time.

An example of this deceit is the myriad pills to treat fever, aches and pains in the marketplace. Such medications will become even more numerous in the future, their diversity limited only by man's imagination. Despite their numbers, however, these pills almost all contain either aspirin or acetaminophen, and some contain both. The *Physicians' Desk Reference for Nonprescription Drugs* lists 43 brands of aspirin and 65 brands of acetaminophen, of which Tylenol is an example. Their producers advertise each as if it were superior, unique, and with fewer side effects than its competitor's identical product.

More golden rules: never take a new drug unless an older and safer medication is ineffective, or you can't take it because of its side effects. Irritating side effects may accompany the newer medication, however, and may be even more intense. Also, never discard a drug that works simply to try a new one. If you change doctors, your new doctor may suggest you try a new medication, which may be identical to your old one, simply to make you think he is more knowledgeable or up-to-date than your previous doctor.

Refuse it if your present medication is effective and free of side effects.

Finally, carefully follow the directions on how to take your medication. If your prescription allows you to decide the dosage and frequency, take the minimum amount necessary to resolve your problem and discard any leftover medication. Do not share it with your pets, since they may not fare as well as you did with it. Without leftovers, you will also be abolishing the universal urge to self-medicate a future disease.

5. If you happen to be female and even think you are pregnant, take no medication unless it is necessary to preserve your life or a bodily function. This is especially important during the first three months of pregnancy, since your unborn child will share the drug with you. As he or she will be developing the heart, brain, and other organs during this time, the drug, (including alcohol and cigarettes), may interfere with their correct formation.

It can be difficult to know which birth defects are caused by medication and which occur randomly, since up to 4% of all newborns have minor abnormalities. Yet, in the case of the thalidomide tragedy years ago, there was little problem identifying the culprit. According to J.M. Manson, the children whose mothers took the tranquilizer during pregnancy risked severe fetal abnormalities, including: amelia (absence of limbs), phocomelia (short limbs), hypoplasticity of the bones, absence of bones, external ear abnormalities (including anotia, micro pinna, small or absent external auditory canals), facial palsy, eye abnormalities (anophthalmos, microphthalmos), and congenital heart defects. Alimentary tract, urinary tract, and genital malformations have also been documented.

R.W. Smithels and C.G. Newman reported mortality due to thalidomide at or shortly after birth to be about 40%. The damage left a negative imprint on the medical profession that will remain for many years to come.

Since few pregnant women volunteer to join a test group to discover what the effects an experimental drug will have on their unborn child, most are sold with a warning similar to this:

> Reproduction studies have been performed in mice and rats at doses up to "Y" times the human dose and have revealed no evidence of impaired fertility or harm to the fetus due to 'X'. There are, however, no satisfactory and well-controlled studies in pregnant women. Because animal reproductive studies are not always predictive of human response, this drug should be used during pregnancy only if clearly needed.

This is good news if you're a female rat, but not so good if you're not. If a medication will not harm a fetus, it will not harm an adult. The opposite is not true. An effective way to avoid unnecessary medication is to fake pregnancy, at least until your late forties. In today's litigious society, doctors will think twice before prescribing anything for a pregnant woman. What they do prescribe will have been carefully evaluated and documented in the medical literature as being acceptable for use during pregnancy. Therefore, if your doctor thinks you're pregnant and is so concerned about your survival that he feels you need medication, he will suggest one he knows is safe. Now you can check your "wallet calendar" and exclaim you didn't miss your period. You'll both be relieved by the news.

If this false pregnancy excuse appears exaggerated or whimsical, it is not. There is a serious and growing problem in medicine today because of the use of drugs that are many times more damaging to your health than anything from the beginning of recorded history to the beginning of the 21st Century. Protecting your health means more than simply entrusting it to someone else, since if a doctor's main concern (his bank account) does not match yours (a prompt, inexpensive return to former health), he will not hesitate to prescribe unnecessarily.

Explaining why you do not need medication is time-consuming, especially if you're begging for one; writing a prescription is not.

Nursing mothers should heed the same advice about avoiding unnecessary medications. Many drugs are excreted in breast milk, and, even if you are hypertensive, your two week-old infant does not need his blood pressure lowered. If you must take medication, stop nursing unless you are certain it is safe to take it and nurse at the same time.

6. The antibiotic era began in 1928, when Sir Alexander Fleming discovered that the growth of a pus producing bacterium, *Staphylococcus aureus*, disappeared from the area where a green mold was growing. Since the mold was a species of *penicillium*, he called the antibiotic penicillin.

Attempts to use substances derived from one organism to kill another began at least 2500 years ago, when the Chinese used a moldy curd of soybeans to treat boils, carbuncles, and similar infections.

Most people know antibiotics combat bacterial infections, but they take them incorrectly because they do not follow the treatment schedule, or because they take them to treat symptoms or diseases that do not need them, such as a fever or the flu. A doctor I know who indiscriminately prescribed antibiotics for fever agreed they were unnecessary, but he told me he routinely prescribed them for all his patients because, "If I don't prescribe what they want, they'll go elsewhere."

The trend today is for doctors to over-prescribe medications, making it difficult for a competent doctor to convince a patient he can recover without them.

"Dr. Smith told me aspirin and orange juice will do the

job," the disgruntled patient says to a friend. "But they're too slow. I decided I needed an antibiotic, and since he wouldn't give me a shot, I went to Dr. Brown who did."

This patient will recover despite his unnecessary and possibly dangerous therapy, (antibiotics can create resistant and deadly bacteria), but his honest doctor has lost him to an unscrupulous businessperson.

If you do need an antibiotic, follow the directions on the label carefully, and do not stop after two doses simply because you feel better.

7. Avoid tranquilizers. They account for 12 to 20% of all prescriptions, which is not surprising when one considers how stressful our lives can be at times. Unfortunately, these medications have created a world of socially acceptable junkies, as well as a double standard; it is not uncommon for a Valium popping parent to tell his son it's unhealthy to smoke marijuana.

Tranquilizers perform a chemical lobotomy, allowing the addict to yawn contentedly as his life slips by. They do not solve his problems, they do not positively change his mental status, and in fact they can worsen an underlying, undiagnosed, depression. Doctors prescribe them because it takes minutes to write a prescription, decreasing the time and effort they must expend to help their patients resolve their problems.

In the case of over-activity, a doctor may treat a child with stimulants or tranquilizers, similar to the "soma" in Aldous Huxley's *Brave New World*, until he becomes a model acceptable to his teacher or parents. Discovering that school bores him, or that his teacher's personal problems are influencing the way he performs his job, takes time and is unprofitable. The era of chemical manipulation of the brain has arrived. Any individual at any age who deviates from the herd is a candidate for therapy, even though we know that some of these drugs punch holes in the brains of laboratory animals, and by association, the brains of children, who have taken them for extended periods of time.

While the law punishes those who prescribe tranquilizers without performing a prior history and physical, any doctor who prescribes them simply because his patient seeks them violates the Hippocratic Oath. This states in part:

> The regimen I adopt shall be for the benefit of my patients according to my ability and judgment, and not for their hurt or for any wrong. I will give no deadly drug to any, though it be asked of me, nor will I counsel such.

Sedatives, the tranquilizer's unhealthy sisters, are often prescribed for the elderly who do not sleep well, even though they have less need for sleep (three to six hours is the rule) than young adults. Slower vital functions accompany advanced age, and while a young person may clear 30 milligrams of a sedative from his body before he takes the next dose the following night, Grandma may not eliminate five milligrams in the same period of time.

Therefore each new dose she takes will add to the amount remaining in her body from her last dose until she is in a state of permanent confusion. When this occurs, her doctor may think she had a stroke and hospitalize her. The poor woman, now off her medication, is disoriented and belligerent when she awakens from her narcosis in the middle of the night and finds herself in strange surroundings. The cure? More drugs to calm her.

When I was in practice in Italy, I made a house call on an elderly patient just released from the hospital following an alleged stroke. Yet he showed no signs of having had one. A careful history revealed he had taken a newly pre-scribed sedative before going to the basement to check the heater. The medication kicked in on his way back up the stairs, and he sat down and fell asleep. A family member could not arouse him and called an ambulance. The doctors in the hospital couldn't arouse him either, and diagnosed *"un infarto cerebrale,"* a cerebral infarct. I stopped his medication before he had another one.

A revolution is in progress against doctors who indiscriminately prescribe tranquilizers. In Britain, more than 250,000 people who once took Ativan daily have launched a campaign to ban the drug.

The article in London's *Daily Mail* related that "lawyers acting for at least 25 people who claim their lives have been made a 'living hell' after becoming addicted to the widely-used drug are considering taking action against the manufacturers and doctors who prescribe it."

Professor Michael Orme of Liverpool University said: "I have spoken to patients who said it is more unpleasant to come off Ativan than heroin. I regard both as drugs of addiction. I would say dependency is equally bad."

Wyeth Laboratories has defended Ativan's record, claiming it was safe if prescribed in short doses. They also stated in the PDR, "the effectiveness of Ativan in long-term use, that is, more than four months, has not been assessed by systemic clinical trials."

Despite its long time on the market (it appeared in Italy in 1972), a company representative, whom I contacted to discuss the case of an elderly patient that had been taking high doses of the drug for three years and was addicted to it, admitted there were no studies available which assessed the drug's long-term use.

8. Therapy is opinion. Even if we understood the biological intricacies of the human body, treating its diseases

would still depend solely on a doctor's judgment and experience. An example is your sore throat. If the cause is viral, gargling warm salt water, standing on your head in the corner, or reading by the light of a flashlight under the covers when you should be asleep, will all cure you in the same amount of time.

If the cause is bacterial, you'll need an antibiotic, but the type and dosage would be at the discretion of your doctor. It would depend on your age, weight, known allergies, and maybe on available free samples in his office if you're poor. Treatment may include ampicillin, penicillin, or erythromycin, in liquid, capsule, or injectable form if you could not swallow.

While most diseases require only brief treatment, others need long-term therapy prescribed in building block form over time until your doctor reaches his desired therapeutic goal. This is where your ignorance creates a problem. A competent doctor, aware of the various therapies in the marketplace, will follow a tried and proven plan and avoid contrasting therapies. For example, his treatment of hypertension will usually begin with diet change, weight loss, exercise, and a diuretic, to which he will gradually add stronger medications until your blood pressure returns to normal. If you are in a hurry to lower it and do not understand the dangers involved in over-treating your disease, you may sabotage his plan.

At the suggestion of a friend with the same problem, you may decide to add his medications to your own to get better results. If your friend's medication is identical to yours but is marketed under a different trade name, adding the two together may increase a safe dose to a toxic one. If his medication is different, there may be a contraindication to take it with yours, and it could result in a serious or life-endangering problem.

Understanding the dosage, side effects and contraindications of medications, especially when they are mixed, is difficult for a professional; to the self-treating uninformed patient it can be deadly. Self-prescribed drugs, or multiple medications prescribed by different doctors without their knowledge, may spell disaster. If your disease does respond to your present therapy, do not change your treatment plan without first consulting your doctor. When in doubt whether to plan your own treatment or not, the best plan is no plan.

Statistics estimated the cost of polypharmacy, or the taking of conflicting medications, at $76.5 billion a year. In the total, the SMART Coalition in California includes hospitalizations at $47.4 billion; long-term care at $14.4 billion; doctor visits at $7.5 billion; emergency department treatment at $5.3 billion; and additional prescriptions at $1.93 billion. Those who died were not included in the totals, neither was the cost of their burials.

9. Make certain the primary purpose of your medication is to treat your primary illness. If you need to take a drug to treat a mild problem and can stop it after a few days, this idea is not especially important. If you need it to treat a lifelong ailment, it will be.

An example is the use of Procardia to treat hypertension. This medication does lower blood pressure, but its main purpose is to treat heart pain, as I discussed in an earlier chapter. If you have high blood pressure and do not have heart disease, this is not a drug for you. You would be better off with a simple water pill, which your doctor should prescribe only after his "back-to-health" advice has proved unsuccessful. This, which I repeat here because of its importance, includes exercise, diet change, cessation of smoking, weight loss, and training in stress reduction.

One way to learn the uses, contraindications, and side

effects of any medication is to read the information sheet that comes with it. Your pharmacist will include it with your prescriptions, and he will discuss your drug with you when you pick it up at his store.

Nowadays you can find information about anything and everything on the Internet, even if some of it will be less factual than you might realize. Even so, if you can, buy a copy of the *Physicians' Desk Reference* (PDR). Even if it is a remainder and does not contain the newest drugs on the market, it is still useful. You will not need information about the newer products unless you have unsuccessfully tried all the older ones. If you do, you should be able to find it on the Internet. If you cannot find your prescribed drug in a year-old PDR, either it has been removed it from the market because it is ineffective, unprofitable, and causes serious side effects, or it is too new for your needs.

The pharmacists' information sheets and the PDR read like a war novel, describing the rashes, itching, bleeding, vomiting, impotence, and even death that indiscriminately strike down victims of the prescription ritual. The abundance of warnings may scare many of you away from taking the medication, which in itself may be good. However, these are symptoms patients like you have experienced while they were taking the medicine in question. It is irrelevant whether they occurred because of an interaction with other medications, unintentional overdosing, or because they would have occurred naturally during the disease. They still occurred.

10. Make sure the drug the pharmacist (or nurse, if you're in the hospital) gives you is the one your doctor ordered. We naturally believe everything prescribed for us will be dispensed correctly, however, pharmacists and nurses can on occasion give us the wrong medication.

While in the hospital you may not know if your nurse

is giving you the right medication, or as is occasionally reported in the newspapers, is poisoning you because he has decided it is time for you to leave your earthly bonds. But if the pill your nurse is giving you looks different from the one you take at home, ask why. It may be the same medication produced by a different company, but it doesn't hurt to check.

At home you can use your *PDR* to verify the pills in the childproof and often adult proof bottle are the ones your doctor prescribed. There is a color guide in its front section that describes all the medications contained in the book. Look up the name of your drug in its pink section, and then go to the color guide. The picture should be identical to the pill in your bottle.

You may face some difficulty if your doctor prescribes a generic drug or a well-known drug and checks the "may substitute" box on your prescription. If he does, the name on the bottle may differ from the one on your prescription. This does not mean the pharmacist can give you birth control pills instead of sleeping pills; it simply allows him to substitute a less expensive drug for the brand name on the script. For example, he can substitute penicillin V, the chemical compound, for Pen Vee K, the trade name of the drug produced by Wyeth-Ayerst Company. Since five or six drug companies produce penicillin V under different names and in different shapes, sizes and colors, you may have to search through the list of penicillin V producers to make sure what your pharmacist gave you is what was prescribed for you.

If your doctor prescribes naproxyn, Pharmacist A may give you Naprosyn by Roche, a white pill with the words "Naprosyn" and "250" stamped on it, and Pharmacist B may give you Naproxyn Tablets, which are green with "N 11" stamped on them. The pills do not look alike but the medication is identical. Your PDR will confirm that the medication, although different in form, color, and size, is the one your doctor prescribed.

Also, beware of pills that look alike but are different, such as Verelan by Lederle and Tetracycline HCl Capsules by Lederle Standard Products. The former is a cardiac drug; the latter an antibiotic. Both are purple and yellow capsules. You do not want to confuse the two.

If you cannot find your pill in the color catalog of the PDR, check the description of the drug in the book's white pages, since not all drugs in the PDR appear in the photo identification section. If you have questions about a medication you think might be in error, be sure to talk to your pharmacist before you take it. If he did give you the wrong medication, he will thank you for bringing it to his attention, especially if he can correct his mistake before your lawyers do.

11. Allopathy (a method of treating disease with remedies that produce effects different from those caused by the disease itself) is what your local doctor practices, but it is not the only theory available. Practitioners of alternative forms of medicine, such as acupuncture, medicina ayurvedica, mesotherapy, homeopathy, or chiropractic, will suggest different treatments for the same disease.

There are many ways to resolve your health problem, from the use of multiple vitamin injections to watered down medications and manipulation, and they may all be correct. Just as two allopathic doctors may suggest different cures to treat your illness, an acupuncturist, a homeopath, a herbalist, or a chiropractor, will suggest different medications and opinions to cure your problem.

The variety of treatments available, as well as your body's tendency to miraculously cure itself after your check arrives for your workman's compensation covered accident, is a source of material for talk shows and newspaper articles. Take all of them with a grain of salt before choosing any of them to cure your ailment.

Since the human body can survive almost all its ills, injuries and their therapies by itself, it is logical the treatments offered by any practitioner will usually be effective. To cite an exotic example, when I worked at an Indian Health Clinic, Shania, a middle-aged woman with diabetes, came to see me for post-nasal drip. I reviewed her chart and found she had not had her insulin and hypoglycemic medications refilled in a long time, even though her last recorded blood sugar was over 400 mg./dl. (normal is below 110 mg./dl.). I asked her if she needed refills, but she said, "No. My medicine man gave me some herbs to take for my sugar. He told me I wouldn't need the shots any more."

She agreed to let me check her blood sugar to see how his therapy was working. It was 78 mg./dl., which is normal. I could not find out which herb her medicine man had given her, but it grew wild somewhere on the Navajo reservation.

This case had a positive ending, but problems may result when traditional healers fail to cure serious diseases and refuse to allow their patients to try other therapies.

Although Shania's case is unusual, it clearly shows there are many ways to cure your illnesses. Unfortunately some of the offers come from charlatans eager to take your money. Before you begin *any* therapy for a chronic disease, please evaluate all your treatment alternatives.

Herbs are fine, and many of our drugs are found in nature, such as digitalis for heart failure, belladonna for eye and intestine aliments, aspirin for aches and pains, and penicillin for infections. These and other ancient remedies are still in use today, although they now may be synthesized in a laboratory instead of cultivated in a garden.

Before placing too much trust in new, expensive, powerful, and dangerous drugs, remember they are more likely to fall by the wayside than the older ones, especially because of the damage they can cause. An example is Redux, the weight loss pill for the markedly obese that was pulled off the market years ago. While guaranteeing only a five-pound weight loss after a year of weight gains and losses, an absurd reason to take the drug, it also guaranteed heart valve damage.

Since a letter I wrote to *The New England Journal of Medicine* years ago regarding the use of Laetrile, a bogus cancer therapy in vogue at the time, applies to all similar therapies, I reproduce it here:

> I am personally opposed to the use of Laetrile, not merely because it is ineffective but also because of the enormous cost, anguish, and ultimate disillusionment it causes its users.
>
> The problem with Laetrile is not simply medical, since it is not employed by reputable physicians, but rather moral or ethical, in that it is incumbent on physicians to protect their patients from fraudulent medication and healers – and often from the patients themselves. Had the medical community in standard testing programs employed this drug, it would have been discarded with little fanfare. But Laetrile has become the drug of hope for the truly desperate whom standard medicine has turned away, and it can only be eliminated when we in orthodox medicine are able to cure all diseases quickly and effectively, or (more probably) when another 'wonder drug' appears on the scene to replace it, touted as the cure-all by hucksters who are

able to capture the media and prey on people's refusal to accept their mortality. Ironically the devil we know may be better than the devil we don't know.

If you decide to experiment with an alternative form of therapy, keep in mind the following:

- Discuss it with your doctor first. He may allow it, but he might know why you should not stop his therapy and switch to a wonder drug.
- Don't take medications from unlabeled bottles or experiment with herbs growing in vacant fields.
- Don't buy medications from the Internet, especially if they're offered in an email from someone who has problems spelling easy words or is selling restricted drugs without a prescription.
- Talk with your doctor or pharmacist before giving OTC (over the counter) medications to the seniors and children in your family, especially if they are taking other medications.
- Leave the medications in their original, labeled bottles and keep them away from children. Telling the emergency room doctor your two year-old took a blue pill from a green bottle you found in a dumpster at a shopping mall will not help him help your comatose child.

12. Despite the advertisements, don't ask your doctor to prescribe a medication you saw on TV or in a magazine! These advertisements by smiling actors that have undergone frontal lobotomies and tout the drug's benefits while rambling quickly over its side effects like auctioneers in a car lot, are meant to make money for the drug companies. If they happen to make you better at the same time, fine. But many ads are misleading (do we really believe that *all*

men over age thirty need Viagra?) and the drugs they peddle often had no purpose until drug companies invented diseases they could "cure" with them. You will not find a medical textbook that describes "erectile dysfunction," "restless legs," or many of the other diseases these companies want you to pester your doctor about.

Your doctor has probably seen the drug advertisements on TV, and if he thought those drugs were good for you, he would prescribe them without your having to ask. Since the drug companies want to sell the products he disapproves of, and since you can't order them yourself without a license, they pressure you directly to convince your doctor to do so.

The fact he will not prescribe them is not because he does not know about them, but because you do not need them. Pressuring him to prescribe them for you will be a disservice to both of you.

I think this is sleazy advertising and should be banned from TV in the United States as it is in the rest of the world, but politics is politics, and there is much more at stake here than your health. The people who come up with these sales pitches have "golden parachutes" and million dollar bonuses to think about.

In summary, never hassle your doctor to prescribe the drugs you hear about on TV. It would be like having your children pressure you into buying an expensive toy you can't afford. You wouldn't, or shouldn't, give in to them, and you shouldn't expect your doctor to give into you either. But if he does without a whimper, he is not one you can trust with your life.

13. Believe in your grandmother's cures. They are not modern, yet they help pass the time, letting the body heal itself. They also cost little and obey the first rule of medicine: *primum non nocere,* "first do no harm." And they are administered with love and concern, the greatest heal-

ing agents known to man. In addition, if Grandma made it to eighty, she must know what she is talking about.

Although the Salernitan guide to health published centuries ago has been quoted so often as to become trite, its suggestion is still appropriate:

> Use three physicians still, first Doctor Quiet,
> Next Doctor Merryman, and Doctor Diet.

The pharmaceutical industry has developed medications that have saved many lives. Unfortunately, some of them, such as DES, the Dalkon Shield, and thalidomide, have taken many others. Medications prescribed inappropriately or unnecessarily compound those tragedies. I cannot stress it enough: *if you are aware of the side effects of your medication and take it only when necessary and as directed, it will work for you, rather than against you.*

Oh, by the way! If you decide to try the egg-fever cure I mentioned at the beginning of this chapter, leave the egg in the shell until it is cooked.

Chapter Six

STOP THE AMBULANCE:
Avoiding Unnecessary Hospitalizations

"I reckon being ill as one of the great plea-
sures of life, provided one is not too ill and is
not obliged to work till one is better."
Samuel Butler, The Way of All Flesh
LXXX.

When Dante Alighieri wrote in the *Divine Comedy*,
"All hope abandon, ye who enter here," he was not referring to a hospital but to hell, although at times the difference between the two is indistinguishable. Skepticism
about your need to be in a hospital to treat your illness will
preserve your health and finances.

Even if public relations agencies work overtime to
convince you their hospitals are "Where Good Things Happen," and Blue Cross once touted, "one American in seven
will be hospitalized (during any year)," the truth is that after prescription drugs, hospitals are the greatest threat to
your health. Statistics show there were 195,000 in-hospital
deaths from medical errors in 2000.

The earliest hospital was in ancient Babylon where the
ill lay on mats in the marketplace and passersby paused to
suggest cures while shopping. As described by Montaigne,

"the whole people was the physician." Today businesspersons have erected buildings in the marketplace, and their mats, once free, now cost hundreds of dollars or more a day. Physician-passersby in the new institutions, sometimes no more informed than the average Babylonian shopper, still poke and probe into their patients' psyche and anatomy, but now their suggestions result in expensive medical or surgical procedures.

Today's hospitals also offer "benefits" of which the Babylonians never dreamed. One is a nosocomial infection, which is caused by bacteria that have lived all their lives in hospitals, thrives on ordinary antibiotics, and claims tens of thousands of lives a year. Powerful drugs, whose cost makes the room rent look like a bargain, can only temporarily tame these germs.

Your doctor should hospitalize you only if you are seriously ill, if he cannot care for you at home or in his office, and if you have a reasonable expectation of recovery. He should not hospitalize you simply because you are dying and your family wants to leave town for a month-long vacation.

If you are in the hospital and are dying, your doctor's discussion with one of your relatives may take the following line:

"Mrs. Jones, your ninety-seven-year-old mother is bleeding internally and her kidneys have failed. She will die if we don't operate."

"But will she survive, Doctor?"

"Does she have insurance?"

"Yes."

"Well, she probably won't, but under the circumstances we should operate anyway."

The "circumstances" relate to her insurance policy and not to her disease. The surgeon would never ask you, the dying patient, directly, since he will not want you to deny him permission to operate. It's much easier for him to make your relatives feel guilty about not doing something that he knows has no possibility of success. After your next-of-kin's consent, sometimes granted by the one who hates you but has the most to inherit, he will bring you to the operating suite, where, despite *his* heroic attempts to snatch you from the jaws of death, *you* fulfill your final destiny.

I have never understood why the patient is never the hero in these scenarios, since he is the one putting his life on the line. Not everything in medicine is logical.

Dying is not un-American and can be done with more dignity at home than elsewhere, as your family's presence can be of great help to you psychologically, emotionally, and physically. Last wishes, blessings, and attempts to resolve past differences are restricted by the sterility of an environment in which you are medicated to the point where any mental faculties you still might possess have disappeared.

Few diseases need to be treated in a hospital, and you can verify this by walking its hallowed halls on a weekend or holiday, and then again the following morning. The increase in the census will astound you.

A fact to ponder: studies show that when hospital based doctors go on strike, a regular event in countries where socialized medicine reigns, *the patient death rate falls by 30-50%*. This is not a coincidence. A patient undergoing needless surgery may die because of the complications of that surgery, but a patient not operated on unnecessarily will not. And a patient that is not getting powerful antibiotics that will make him vulnerable to nosocomial infections by destroying his disease and his resistance at the same time, may improve on his own.

Your doctor may never hospitalize you, but you should

plan for it now rather than wait for the crisis to occur. The following advice is helpful:

1. Avoid hospitalization for anything other than a dire emergency or a voluntary in-house surgical procedure. I strongly discourage voluntary admissions.

In the case of a severe injury or illness, you will need to be hospitalized; in other cases, it may not be so clear. One easy means of resolving the question when you are not feeling ill, is to tell your doctor your spouse has quit his job, your health insurance has lapsed, and you have no cash. If he sends you home, the hospitalization was unnecessary. If he tries to hospitalize you on a later occasion and again changes his mind because of your lack of finances, switch doctors.

This tactic may seem extreme, but if your doctor and hospital think you will not pay them, they will find a less expensive, more practical solution to your problem. In case you doubt the wisdom of pleading poverty, remember it is illegal for a hospital or a doctor to refuse to treat you if your illness or injury is a true emergency. Even Horodotus stated of the Babylonian people-physicians: "And they are not allowed to pass by a sick person in silence, without inquiring the nature of his distemper."

If your doctor insists on hospitalization, even to the unusual extreme of offering free services, his request is probably valid. At this point you can remember your insurance policy does not expire until next month, and agree with him.

Whether his treatment is free or not, you should never be hospitalized for ailments you can treat at home. In the case of a minor problem where it was not necessary, your doctor cannot allow you to lie in bed all day watching soap operas while you wait for your laboratory results to appear on his laptop. He will order round the clock testing to keep your mind preoccupied, and to convince you he is doing something about your problem.

You should also be aware of "Ping-Pong" medicine. This is a moneymaking scheme where *you* are the bouncing ball. Louise, a patient of mine who suffers from migraine headaches, was a victim of this game. She told me her doctor suggested they were due to an unusual form of heart disease and sent her to a cardiologist friend for evaluation. The cardiologist, after performing many expensive tests, found her heart was healthy. However, he thought liver disease might be the cause of her headaches, and hustled her off to his friend, the gastroenterologist.

A neurologist and a rheumatologist also saw Louise before she finally understood their game and broke the cycle.

If you do not understand this ploy, like her you'll bounce from doctor to doctor until all the colleagues in crime have seen you, or until you run out of money or insurance coverage.

As a hospitalized patient, you are a captive participant in this game. Dr. X will have specialists drop by without telling you beforehand. This increases the fear that your problem is serious since so many important specialists have to see you, and it neatly fills the time slot between one unnecessary laboratory test and the next. This is one reason medical bills for even brief admissions run into tens of thousands of dollars.

If you are conscious during your hospitalization, you can avoid this by telling your doctor to ask your permission *before* he sends anyone to see you. If he wants a kidney specialist to evaluate your headache, refuse the offer.

2. Never be hospitalized for tests you can have done in the hospital outpatient department or by a private laboratory.

Unless you are seriously ill and need immediate testing, an outside laboratory can perform all your studies at reduced cost. An example of this is my patient who had a H&H (hemoglobin and hematocrit) blood tests while hospitalized. He was charged $99.50 for *each* of these extremely common, simple tests. I later repeated them both for $1.25.

If you feel well enough to stay home and wait the twenty-four hours it will take to get their results, you should do so. And before you begin a second series, have your doctor explain in detail what he learned from the first reports and why he needs further testing.

Also, if you have agreed to be hospitalized for a non-urgent illness, try to have all your necessary (or unnecessary but required) tests completed *before* your admission. Some hospitals want to perform your tests in their laboratories and will not accept results of tests performed elsewhere, even if they were done the same day.

The reason that your health may have worsened between the brief time you completed your tests and your admission, and this could compromise your health care, even if you are being hospitalized for a benign procedure such as a hernia repair.

This is not the real reason, of course; they are simply looking to increase their profits. Even so, if you need to have your hernia repaired and your hospital refuses to admit you until you have your testing done in its laboratory, ask your physician to schedule you to have them done as an outpatient at the hospital the day before the surgery. He should then admit you only if the results permit surgery. Delay your hospitalization if tests suggest you have a minor problem that would preclude general anesthesia.

Finally, if he cannot admit you on the day of your surgery, never let him hospitalize you more than one day before your non-urgent procedure, nor on a Friday, Saturday or on any holiday for any reason except a true emergency. Since hospitals schedule non-emergency procedures on weekdays, an admission on a holiday will only increase your costs and risks.

3. If you are in a hospital and think you should be elsewhere, you are probably right. Some physicians tend to keep their fully insured patients in the hospital until they can find similar ones to take their places. The number of patients these doctors discharge from the hospital just before they go on vacation is astounding.

If your idea of what your health should be differs from your doctor's, he may refuse your request for release. At this point, you can either accept his opinion and hope he will be going on vacation soon, or press onward. If you do decide to leave, hospital bigwigs will swoop into your room, each offering reasons why you must not leave. If you hold your ground, they will relent, but only after forcing you into signing a form relieving them of any responsibility for your presumed immediate death. At this point, ignore snide comments about how thin and pale you are, or that your surgical wound might reopen.

The best tactic is to be firm but nonviolent. Thank the staff for all they have done for you, remind them you have four young children at home who have not eaten since your hospitalization began, and assure them you will immediately return should your condition worsen. I have yet to see a patient return when he was firmly convinced he no longer belonged in the hospital.

4. Select your hospital while you can still perform basic mathematical functions. Hospitals may someday post their prices by their entrances, which may encourage competition, but until they do, they will continue to charge as much as they can. The next chapter will explain how to evaluate prices; however, the most expensive hospital is the

most expensive, period. You will not get a better quality chest X-ray for $80.00 than you would for $40.00, which is important to remember if you have to pay part or all of your bill yourself.

While selecting your hospital, you should also check its track record. If the Joint Commission on Accreditation of Healthcare Organizations, a private, nonprofit group, has accredited yours, it will send you a free report of its findings, as well as that of its local competitor. This is an easy way to choose the better of the two.

When you've selected the one you think is right for you, the admission clerk will give you a bundle of forms to sign. Read them first. They will include an advanced directive form, where you decide if you want someone pounding on your chest to revive you if you should die during your operation. Other forms allow doctors to take further steps in your treatment based on your presurgical decisions if you're unconscious at the time. For example, you may want your surgeon to remove your breast if your lump turns out to be cancerous. Or you may prefer to have the radical surgery performed later. Whatever you decide you *must* put in writing. The old saying, "If it wasn't written down, it didn't happen," is true in medicine.

Lastly, make sure you understand what all the "ites" and "oses" mean. If you didn't understand your choices and later protest your surgeon's actions, the courts may agree your misunderstanding of the documents contents prevented you from giving informed consent. But this is only a *legal* benefit. The courts cannot give you your breast back if it turns out you did not have cancer and it was removed unnecessarily.

To paraphrase Smokey the Bear, "Only you can prevent unnecessary hospitalizations."

EMERGENCY DEPARTMENTS

Walking through the front door is the conventional way of being admitted to the hospital, but there is a more subtle way of entering the hallowed halls of healing: through the emergency department (ED).

The ED (also known as the ER) is a place to get care quickly, but not if you do not have a life-threatening injury or disease. It is not run as a bakery, with each client being served in strict numeric rotation, nor should it be.

Major injuries and illnesses take precedence over minor ones, and even if you think your pneumonia is important, the staff will ignore you until they have treated all the true emergencies. Also, it would be unusual if your problem did not need laboratory and X-ray studies; these also are performed after the genuine emergencies are out of the way. Therefore, before you see the doctor, you will have to wait until the real casualties have been treated; if any more arrive before your turn comes, you again go to the back of the line. Under this system, you may recover from your illness before you are discharged from the ED.

A word of warning: *Emergency departments are for emergencies only*. Do not go to your local ED unless your problem is life threatening or will result in severe or permanent damage if it is not treated within twenty-four hours. Even then, I strongly suggest you contact your doctor first, and go to your ED only if he is unavailable and does not have a colleague covering for him, an unlikely and possibly illegal situation.

If your have a true emergency and an ambulance or your friends have brought you to the ED, ask to have your doctor treat you. Even if you will not save a dime on the cost of your care, you are better off if a doctor who knows your health problems treats you. As an unbelievable but true example of what can happen if you don't, a nurse told me her hospital director could not find a qualified ED doctor to work in his small-town emergency room one Christmas, so he hired a chiropractor for the day. Can you imagine the effect his spinal manipulation of your spine would have had on your heart attack?

Although you can benefit from your ED under the right circumstances, your uneducated use of the facility can be costly and dangerous. You should remember the following points:

1. Before you need aid, ask if your hospital has neurosurgeons, cardiac surgeons, ophthalmologists, and orthopedic surgeons on its staff. You can get a copy of the hospital's roster of doctors and their specialties from it's administrator. If no specialists are available (as in an Urgent Care Center posing as an Emergency Department), call the larger hospitals in your area until you find one that has these doctors, as you will need them if you hope to survive your more serious problems.

To avoid the wiles of a small hospital impersonating a major medical center, check the office addresses of all the specialists who are on its list of providers. Many of them will have never been inside your hospital, and may live many miles away from your area. They have privileges there simply in case they might need to see a patient in your local hospital someday. For a specialist to be useful, he must be nearby, since even doctors find it difficult to be in two places at once.

You can discover your hospital's capabilities by asking what its emergency room rating is. A hospital with a level one or two trauma center means it can handle all emergencies on a 24-hour basis; a level four is a first aid station. A small, private, fee-for-service hospital providing level four care will usually have a doctor on duty (I hope not a chiropractor) who will not be trained to treat major emergencies. Thus, if you have a leaking aortic aneurysm, a tear in the lining of the main artery of the body that will create heirs shortly after it ruptures, an ED which offers only basic care, is the last place you would want to be, and the last place you will be.

Moonlighters, or doctors seeking to earn extra dollars while in training or while building a practice, often work in these small hospital emergency rooms. Some of them are ill suited for the position, but even if you have been lucky enough to find one competent to treat your problem, you still may need a specialist to complete your care. Therefore, it is better to travel thirty miles to a hospital offering major emergency services, than to race to a local hospital to be treated for your aneurysm by a moonlighting pediatrician. Since aortic aneurysms are not a cause of death among children, he will have no experience in treating yours, if he can even diagnose it.

Make sure you tell all your family members where you want them to take you for serious health problems.

2. Going to the ED of a teaching or voluntary hospital may result in admission to the hospital for many reasons, most of which will not involve money. Going to a private, investor-owned hospital's ED may also result in an admission for many reasons, most of which will involve money.

Teaching hospitals are not sin-free, however, as they must keep a daily patient quota to maintain their rating. When that falls below a certain level, program directors send orders to the ED to admit "X" number of patients. If your ED doctor suggests admission to the hospital, make sure it is not merely to fill an empty teaching bed. You can do this by carefully triaging your ED to your needs, and specifically:

For all life-threatening emergencies, your best choice

is a teaching hospital with a level one or two ED. The important factor here is the immediate availability of specialists.

For a minor illness or injury the above may still be your best choice. There is one drawback: you may not avoid an unnecessary hospitalization here by pleading poverty, since a social worker will get you a card entitling you to free everything, whether you deserve it or not. And then if a subsequent search through computer records reveals you do have insurance, you'll find yourself in an awkward position.

If you do have insurance, but still wish to use the no-insurance ploy to avoid hospitalization for your minor ailment until Grandma returns from her skiing trip in Switzerland, pleading total poverty at a private, for-profit, non-teaching hospital emergency room or a medicenter, described below, is the answer. These are not ideal places to get non-urgent care, but your plea will guarantee you will not be admitted unnecessarily.

The last place an admittedly insured patient with a minor problem, or a patient with a major health problem and a choice, should seek help is at a private, for-profit, hospital offering only basic emergency services. This is an expensive version of your private doctor's office, an opening into the depths of an unhealthy world of economic spoliation that is stranger than fiction.

MEDICENTERS

Any profitable venture has its imitators, and with the excuse that ED costs are too high, businessmen-physicians have invented their own system of heath care delivery. It has various names, but is known as a medicenter or an Urgent Care Center. Californians euphemistically refer to this as "Doc in the Box" medical care.

These mini medical centers, no more equipped than your doctor's office, close at midnight since the graveyard shift (no pun intended) is the least economically profitable. In addition, full moons spawn bizarre acts of aggression whose victims may need hospitalization these centers cannot provide.

While you won't risk unnecessary hospitalization in a medicenter, its philosophical purpose is identical with the ED that offers basic services: to perform as many tests as possible and then refer you to your own doctor for follow-up care. Most medicenters advertise they do not want regular patients, but if you do not have a doctor, they, as the ED, will suggest one from a list of doctors who has signed on to handle such situations. This will result in added fees and tests, since, in the mind of your new doctor, your disease could have changed since your discharge from the medicenter.

It is difficult to assess the value of these centers, and you may not save money by going to them. In a letter to a California newspaper, a disgruntled patient once complained that a medicenter charged him $400.00 to suture a minor cut on his leg. He asserted his local ED would have charged less than half as much for the same service.

While your choices are many, the best is to find a competent general or family practitioner and to remain loyal to him. If he is unavailable and has no substitute, the next best choice for treatment for an acute, but non life-threatening illness, would be a medicenter, since there would be no possibility of unnecessary hospitalization.

Chapter Seven

DON'T BREAK THE BANK:
Spending Your Health Dollars Wisely

"He's a fool that makes his doctor his
heir."
Ben Franklin

If you aren't lucky enough to pass through life without ever being ill, your doctor will someday order expensive blood panels, X-rays, and scans to diagnose your disease and "to rule out…." he'll cryptically say, a more serious ailment. To avoid this costly and sometimes dangerous situation, you will need to find a doctor who can diagnose your ailment simply, inexpensively, and with few, if any, laboratory tests.

If you don't, your self-interested doctor may offer to run his unnecessary tests right in his office, with little preparation, fuss or bother. If he doesn't have an office laboratory, he may send you to a facility with which he may be financially affiliated. Lastly, he may suggest hospitalization so he can perform the procedures more conveniently (for him).

If he suggests the first alternative, immediate testing in his office, he may tell you that you do not need to fast, to save your urine for 24 hours, or to do whatever another patient would need to do if the tests are to be performed correctly and give valid results. If your problem is serious, have them done. But if you don't feel ill, ask him why you don't need to fast when you brother, mother, and pet dog, did when they had the same tests done elsewhere.

If you are timid and prefer to avoid confrontations, simply thank him for his concern and have him print on his prescription pad the name of your disease, the tests he wants, and what he will charge you to perform them in his office. Since some blood tests should be performed only while you are fasting, tell him the two candy bars, four eggs, and the pound of greasy bacon you ate thirty minutes before coming to his office will affect the results and you'd rather wait. Don't forget to add that if he does them immediately, he'll have to repeat them when you are fasting to make sure you do not have high cholesterol, diabetes, or whatever other disease they will suggest, and you can't afford the double expense.

You might even want to warn him that you had a grand-mal seizure the last time you had blood drawn. No doctor likes to have a patient seize in his office.

If your problem is not an emergency, your doctor should agree with you and schedule your tests for the following morning. If not, tell him your best friend is the president of a medical society in another state, and he told you that having routine blood tests performed when you are not fasting is useless. It'll stop him dead in his tracks. It is always to your advantage to have another doctor on your side, especially one with titles, even if he is a phantom.

Now that you've avoided testing, at least temporarily, take your prescription home and open the textbooks I described in chapter four. By now, you know that if the tests your doctor requested have nothing in common with those your textbook recommends to confirm his diagnosis, you are wasting your time and money by having them done. If your symptoms do not even agree with those of the disease your doctor suspects, you have two choices: you can return to him and ask for an explanation, or more practically, simply change doctors. If his diagnosis was that far off the mark, a heated discussion would prove valueless.

If what he asks is appropriate, call the medical and X-ray laboratories in your area and ask how much your tests will cost. If your doctor matches or beats his competition, have him perform the studies. If his charges exceed his competitors', take your prescription to the less expensive laboratory and have the tests done there. And be sure to tell your doctor and all your friends and acquaintances why you did; it may persuade him to lower his prices.

While there is nothing inherently wrong with a doctor testing you in his office, a conflict of interest and a possibility of a technically inferior result do exist. An SMA-12 (jargon for a panel of 12 analyses performed on a small sample of your blood) is not performed on an inexpensive machine like typewriter that uses paper and ribbons. It is expensive and uses a different reagent to perform each of its 12 blood tests, as indicated by its name. If the reagents are outdated, they may not yield accurate results. Therefore, to avoid discarding them and the resulting economic loss, or to use them, risking inaccurate results, an unscrupulous doctor may order all the tests his machine can perform on each patient he sees. This is a reason you may undergo a blood or urine test at each office visit.

While doctors must be certified before taking X-rays in their offices, a significant percentage of the studies performed by those who are not radiologists are of poor quality or even technically useless. Even when they are acceptable, the radiological training of some is so poor they cannot interpret them.

Since the cost of a small X-ray machine runs into tens of thousands of dollars, to recoup its cost, some doctors X-ray every patient with a bruise, cough or hangnail, "just to be sure." If your textbook says an X-ray is necessary, whenever possible have it performed by a radiologist who will perform it correctly and interpret it accurately. This will at least guarantee you get good value for your hard earned money.

If your doctor wants to schedule your tests at a private laboratory or the hospital outpatient laboratory, the same advice to shop around applies. Kickbacks occur in medicine, and the *Wall Street Journal* once reported that charges for laboratory fees were "running at more than $11 billion a year...(and) $1 billion of the total figure reflect(ed) kickbacks and other lab abuses."

Improperly performed examinations are less likely to occur in a reputable laboratory. Since it will perform many analyses per day, it also can offer them at a lower price.

A fact to remember: you cannot buy a better urinalysis or blood test for more money. State regulatory agencies guarantee accuracy by requiring laboratories to undergo quarterly testing and maintain minimum standards. Therefore, your test results should be accurate, regardless of their cost. A laboratory that charges less than its competitor does not necessarily perform inferior work, but if it does not have a certificate on the wall certifying it undergoes periodic testing, search for one that does.

Beware of hospitalization for a few days so that your tests can be run more conveniently! If you have no insurance and no visible means of support, your doctor will not suggest this. If you pay your own bills, refuse this invitation, since it can increase your costs by 10% or more.

If you do need to have your tests performed in a hospital, check into its pricing philosophy beforehand, since luxuries such as a water glass and a disposable pillow can add $1,200.00 a day to your bill.

Economists use the prices of a selected number of common items to monitor inflation, and a "lab basket" will work equally well in helping you discover the pricing strategy of the hospitals in your area. Should there be only one in a 200 mile radius, it will make little difference what it charges. However, if you have a choice and want to know where to find the lowest prices, call the billing offices of all the hospitals in your area and ask what they charge for the following items: daily room charge, chest X-ray, urinalysis, electrocardiogram, SMA-12, and arterial blood gases.

You do not need to know what these tests are, nor whether you will need any of them. Once you have their prices, just add them up to find out which hospital is the most expensive.

If a chest X-ray costs $10.00 more in one hospital than in another, you can be sure a stomach X-ray in that hospital will also cost more. In fact, if the few tests you have asked about at hospital A are more expensive than those at hospital B, then it is probable that all the other tests at hospital A will be more expensive than at hospital B.

Besides the costs of the tests themselves, you need to know if there are drawing or handling fees, or if late fees are added after a certain hour. In some cases, the hospital includes these charges in the price of the tests; in others, they can equal or even exceed it, adding a substantial amount to your overall costs. For example, the hospital may add a $15.00 drawing fee to all blood examinations. Therefore, if the test alone costs $15.00, with the drawing fee it will cost $30.00. If there is a late fee of $20.00 on all tests performed after 8:00 p.m., your test will now cost $50.00. In this case, the cost increased almost fourfold because of arbitrary drawing charges and fees, and knowing the price of the test alone was not enough to make an informed choice.

You also need to ask if the charges are different if you are a patient in the ED, an outpatient, or an inpatient in the hospital. Outpatient service means your doctor schedules a test for you in the hospital, and after you have it performed, you return home and await its results. Inpatient service means you undergo testing while you are a patient in the hospital.

Enrico suffered from ulcer symptoms for many months before his doctor admitted him to his hospital for an X-ray. He paid the $170.00 cost of the procedure, plus $100.00 to the radiologist who read the X-ray. He was later enraged to learn his hospital charged an all-inclusive fee of *$98.00* for the *same* X-ray if its radiologists performed it on an *outpatient*. He learned too late his hospital, in addition to his room costs, had charged him $172.00 more for his X-ray simply because he was a patient *in* the hospital.

Was there a difference between the two procedures? No. The hospital had wanted him as a client, so it advertised low prices. However, when he became an inpatient, he also became a victim of its pricing scam.

The cost difference of the other studies on outpatients and inpatients in this particular hospital was similar, even though their performance was the same in all other respects. The prices it quoted to inquiring patients always were for outpatient studies, although it never explained this to them, and charged them higher rates when they were admitted. The hospital also used its outpatient prices in its advertising, claiming its charges were lower than its competitor's.

If you had been admitted to that hospital and expected the lower charges, would you have been outraged when you received your bill?

This hospital followed the same pricing strategies in its laboratory. When I did this survey many years ago, an outpatient paid $17.50 for the SMA-12 panel at the above institution. Inpatients paid $48.00, and because of late fees, paid $69.00 if they had it done after 8:00 p.m.

To put these charges in perspective, a well-known laboratory chain at the time charged $7.95 for a SMA-24 (24 is the number of blood analyses in the panel). It supplied its doctor affiliates with the equipment they needed to collect and prepare the samples. Since it was located far from the towns it served, couriers collected the specimens and flew them to the laboratory for processing. I'm not praising this particular company, but only explaining that despite its significantly greater overhead, it still made enough profit charging reasonable prices to stay in business.

With far less overhead than its competitor, the hospital charged 220% more for half the number of analyses. When calculated on a one for one basis, it charged its hospitalized patients 1,200% more. And it charged an astounding 1,735% more than the outside laboratory if it performed the tests after 8:00 p.m.!

My survey of charges in a city thirty miles away, where five hospitals competed for the same patient, showed inpatient and outpatient laboratory charges were identical. One hospital did add a late fee only on procedures performed on outpatients after 11:00 p.m. It was half that of the small-town hospital.

Another survey I made of the charges of country and city hospitals years ago, when prices were more reasonable, (were they ever?), showed the following:

110

Hospital	A	B
Emergency Room charges:	$44.00	$36.25
Chest X-ray, 2 views:	$56.00	$57.00
(Outpatient:	**$40.00)**	
Electrocardiogram:	$55.00	$50.00
Urinalysis:	$12.00	$9.50
(Outpatient:	**$5.00)**	
SMA-12	$48.00	$47.25
(Outpatient:	**$17.50)**	
Arterial Blood gases	$76.00	$40.00
Late fees after 8:00 p.m.		
Laboratory	$22.00	$00.00
X-ray	$19.00	$00.00
Late fees after 11:00 p.m.	As above	$11.00
Total ED charges with clinical analyses:		
After 8:00 p.m.	$332.00	$240.25
After 11:00 p.m.	$332.00	$251.25

The dollar figures in boldface are what you would have paid to have your tests performed as an outpatient in hospital A. If your doctor had ordered a chest X-ray ($40.00), urinalysis ($5.00) and an SMA-12 ($17.50) for you as an outpatient in that hospital, you would have spent $62.50. As a patient in its ED you would have paid $109.00, and you would have paid $150.00 if you arrived after 8:00 p.m.

If your insurance company pays your medical bills, these statistics may not interest you. However, if your budget is stretched to the limit and you must pay a large deductible or your entire bill, you will appreciate the 25%

savings you can get if your doctor treats you in the ED of voluntary hospital B instead of privately owned hospital A. You will save even more, 60% to be exact, if you have your non-emergency tests performed as an outpatient before 8:00 p.m.

This is only one example of the many ways hospitals overcharge their patients. If you are a wise shopper, you will save money.

If you have chosen your doctor carefully, and have followed all my rules to avoid unnecessary medication and laboratory analyses, but had to be hospitalized because of a serious illness, be sure to review your hospital and medical bills carefully before you pay them. I had a patient who had a cast put on his broken wrist; his hospital bill included $700.00 for a hip prosthesis.

Another bait-and-switch ploy is the "phantom panel." Your doctor may order an SMA-12 panel, traditionally an inexpensive way of ordering blood tests, but the hospital's billing office may charge for each of the 12 tests as if he had ordered them individually. You will receive a bill for $160.00 instead of the $20.00 they advertised and you expected.

Insurance companies understand this tactic, routinely recombine the tests into panel format, and then reduce the charges. While you may not be able to do this on your own, if you believe this has occurred, have your doctor review your bill with you. It should be easy for him to correct his hospital's billing "error."

Another example of aggressive billing is that of a patient who needed simple inter-hospital transportation. She was in no distress and received no medical attention during the $440.00, 35 mile trip. Since the ambulance company would not discuss her bill either with her or me, I contacted her insurance company. They found the company had submitted a bill for $430.00, not the $440.00 it had billed the patient, the extra charge for emergency transportation was unwarranted, and the mileage charge was excessive. Because of the patient's curiosity and tenacity, she succeeded in reducing her charges by 22% or $95.00. Needless to say, the ambulance company was not overjoyed by the change.

Even if insurance companies reduce some of the more outrageous bills, hospital costs are still many times what they need to be. The fleam, a primitive surgical knife used for bloodletting, has been resurrected as today's medical bill.

Caveat emptor.

Chapter Eight

EXTEND YOUR WARRANTY:
Protecting Your Long Term Health

"Tiberius was wont to mock at the arts of physicians, and at those who, after thirty years of age, needed counsel as to what was good or bad for their bodies."
Plutarch: <u>Morals</u>, p. 514.

Much has been said about the use of modern technology to prevent illness, but the truth behind the hyperbole is that apart from some infectious diseases, medical science can *prevent* very few maladies. A doctor cannot prevent diabetes by examining your urine for sugar once a month, nor can he prevent lung cancer by performing a yearly chest X-ray. In the latter disease, the success rate of early detection in heavy smokers is so dismal the American Cancer Society no longer suggests it. According to a report from the Medical College of Pennsylvania, a group of six-thousand males screened with chest X-rays every six months for ten years had the same death rate from lung cancer as did the unscreened population.

An even more disappointing study shows 25% of lung cancers discovered on X-ray after patients became symptomatic with them had been present on earlier X-rays, but had been missed by the radiologists who had reviewed them.

The best preventive medicine technique to avoid lung cancer is to quit smoking and to avoid inhaling toxic substances, such as asbestos, in your home or workplace.

Laboratory testing doesn't fare much better since statistics show that 7% to 12% of all results are in error. This means you have about a one in ten chance of being diagnosed as having a disease you do not have, and the same chance of not being diagnosed with the one you do have. A misdiagnosis that ruined one patient's day was cancer of the prostate, a disease that belonged to the patient ahead of him that was given a clean bill of health.

I once questioned the results of a urinalysis I was certain was wrong. The technician told me the results of the automated testing passed through three different computers before being printed. The first computer performed the test, the second computer collected the results, and the third printed them on a lab slip. Because of a technical glitch, this last computer was matching the results from the first test of the day to the name of the last patient who had been tested the day before, even though his name should have been cleared from the list. Every patient that day got the test results of the person following him in line.

If you have noticed a recent change in some bodily function, don't think it's unimportant just because all your tests were normal a month ago. A change in health is a change in health, period. No doctor can order all the tests available in today's market, and even if he could, they would reflect only your present health. None is accurate enough to find the artery in your head that will rupture when your blood pressure exceeds its limit of tolerance, or the stone in your kidney that will move and cause pain.

And there is no test he can order that will detect cancerous changes in a few intestinal cells when the disease is curable. An example of the unreliability of a routine physical is the tumor nesting in the colon of an ex-President of the United States. He had access to the best specialists in the country and underwent yearly intestinal examinations, yet his doctors *did not find his cancer until after it had been present for several years.*

If you are healthy and vigorous with no symptoms of illness, you do not need a yearly physical, as the likelihood of discovering an unsuspected disease is almost nonexistent. A study at the Permanente Medical Group of over 10,000 patients aged between 35 and 54 agrees that periodic health examinations have little impact on overall health status.

Critics of managed care plans complain this and similar data are being used to provide fewer and less comprehensive check-ups, but they don't realize in medicine, less is often more. Routine testing is rarely productive and can be dangerous if it extends to routine angiograms for possible heart disease, and routine surgical interventions for mole and bump removal.

I know of a young woman who had a "bump" removed from the angle of her jaw. Her surgeon also removed a piece of her facial nerve at no extra charge, leaving her with a total paralysis of one half of her face.

On the positive side, instead of relying on medicine to prolong your life, you can do so yourself by changing some of your peskier habits, such as drinking, smoking, and drug abuse. Alcoholism is now being diagnosed as a hereditary disease, and I imagine smoking will soon follow. I believe they are simply bad habits that lead to health problems. We know smokers risk chronic bronchitis, emphysema, cancer, mattress fires, and shoot-outs in restaurants when they offend the sensibilities of a non-smoker dining at a nearby table.

While smoking has no redeeming value other than to make you feel grown-up at a party, drinking is a different problem. Some reports show people who drank heavily and then quit run a greater risk of early death from heart attacks than those who simply cut back on their consumption. Other reports suggest that people who have one or two drinks a day live longer than people who have never imbibed. These reports are put out by the wine industry.

No one knows how much alcohol is safe, but if your drinking results in blackouts or affects the way you perform your job or your relationship with family members, you are drinking too much.

Environment is also an important determinant in the health game. If you live in the Love Canal, a working-class neighborhood near Niagara Falls built on tons of chemical waste, you'll not need to wonder where you will spend your retirement checks.

The best advice I can give you about your use of medicine's modern miracles is to pay close, but not exaggerated, attention to your body. When it starts performing erratically, find out why. A day old cough without other symptoms does not need medical attention; one lasting six months with fever, weight loss, and blood in your phlegm does.

If you have recently begun having chest pains and underwent a physical a month ago, do not rely on its glowing results as proof they are unimportant, and don't await your next physical before seeking help, since you may not live that long. More than one patient has suffered a heart attack minutes after being told his ECG was normal.

Regarding preventive medicine schemes, proponents of the yearly physical examination traditionally divide their patients into two classes based on their wealth and social standing, one meriting more preventive care than the other. One doctor I know performs simple, routine blood tests on his poor patients. His insured business executives, however, get X-rays of their stomachs, kidneys, and gallbladders. And "just to be sure," he repeats them every two years for as long as his patients have health insurance.

Gallstones afflict one in five people throughout the world, unless you are a female Pima Indian from southern Arizona, where the incidence is seven in ten. Even so, this doctor is concerned about more about his welfare than his patients' health when he irradiates their gallbladders every 24 months. Even if they have gallstones, there is no need to treat them unless they cause symptoms.

Some doctors also suggest patients get a limited number of inexpensive procedures regularly, although they disagree about which ones to order and how often to run them. Many times, they base their test selection simply on their availability in a local laboratory.

If, in spite of my warnings, you still wish to be part of this group, a logical preventive program should consider your age, be it infancy or advanced age, even if neither is preventable.

Your child, not a pint-sized adult but an individual with specific needs, will need frequent doctor visits only in his first year of life. His initial checkup should be in the delivery room, and if performed correctly, will uncover most of his physical defects present at birth. The remaining three or four visits during his first year serve simply to evaluate his growth and development and to vaccinate him against some of yesterday's plagues, including polio, diphtheria, and tetanus.

In his second year, the frequency of his checkups should decrease precipitously if he is healthy. One examination before entering school to bring his vaccinations up-to-date, and two or three more check-ups before the teenage years should be enough. This schedule refers only to well-child care, of course, and not to the frequency with which a doctor should see an ill child.

Pediatricians, in fierce competition with family practitioners for the ever-dwindling pool of patients, are now reluctant to release their charges until they replace them with their progeny. As a result, some have introduced routine, adult style laboratory tests into their practice. The likelihood of finding a disease in a healthy, active, bright child is as dismal as finding one in a healthy adult, and I would not test them routinely.

However, discussion of an unconventional life-style which includes drugs, poor nutrition, and promiscuous sex, is in order at any age.

Vaccinations can prevent many childhood diseases, yet they themselves can cause problems, and some parents refuse to have their children vaccinated. Most states have taken the option out of the hands of parents and doctors.

Our body has an immune system that exists to defend us from microscopic organisms that can harm or kill us. Drug companies are of the opinion that they know more than our immune systems do about protecting us, and have invented vaccines, some of which in my opinion, serve little or no purpose. In addition, to sell their products they will sometimes use "statistics" that are misleading. Stating that the shingles vaccine will reduced your likelihood of catching the disease in later life by 50% is true. However, statistically only 1.7 people out of every 100 will suffer from it. Among the vaccinated, 0.8% will. Since I've never seen 8/10 of a person walking the streets, the odds of catching the disease are about the same in the vaccinated and the unvaccinated population.

Since the 1940s the number of vaccinations the CDC

recommends (not requires) for 18 year-olds and under has increased six-fold. Only one, smallpox, has been eliminated from the list.

Late 1940s

Smallpox	Tetanus
Diphtheria	Pertussis

Late 1970s

Diphtheria	Measles
Tetanus	Mumps
Pertussis	Rubella
Polio(OPV)	

2023

Diphtheria	Polio(IPV)
Tetanus	Hib
Pertussis	HepatitisB
Measles	Varicella
Mumps	HepatitisA
Rubella	Pneumococcal
Meningococcal ACWY	Influenza
Meningococcal B	Rotavirus
Humanpapillomavirus	Dengue
Covid-19	

According to the CDC recommended immunization schedule, children and young adults will receive about 40 vaccinations before age 18.

While the producers of these vaccines disagree that their cash cows might be contributing to the staggering increase in autism in the youth of the world, statistics show that in the 60s and 70s only two to four children in 10,000 were autistic.

The chart below shows the number of cases of autism from 1975 (1:5000) to 2009 (1:110). In 2018, according to the CDC, the ratio had increased dramatically to 1:44 (Autism Spectrum Disorder -ASD).

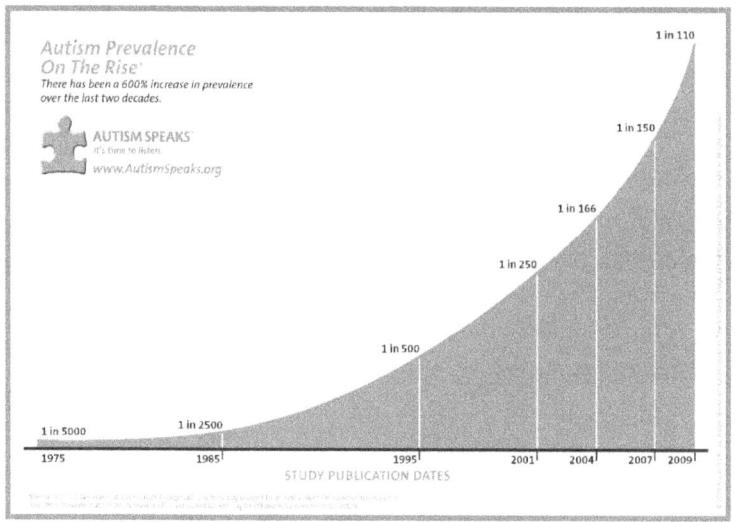

The following vaccines have been around for a while and deserve mentioning:

1. DPT: This anagram, in many versions, is the vaccination against Diphtheria, Pertussis, and Tetanus. Diphtheria does not have a nickname I am aware of, but the others are known as "whooping cough" and "lockjaw." The series of vaccinations begins in the second month of life and is completed when the child enters school. After age six the pertussis vaccine is dropped from the trio. Everyone should get a tetanus booster every ten years, more often only in the case of a severely contaminated wound.

2. TOPV, or trivalent oral polio vaccine, is usually

121

given with the DPT vaccine. It replaced my Mother's advice to "rest during the hot summer afternoons," and not to "play near the garbage can," as prevention of polio.

3. MMR or Measles-Mumps-Rubella, is the last major vaccination worth noting now that science has eradicated smallpox. The vaccination for the pox is not given any longer, but reports that AIDS became a problem only after an extensive vaccination program against the pox in Africa marred the celebration of the last known case of the disease.

There was a significant drop in the number of reported measles cases after the introduction of MMR, but epidemics still occur. One of the presumed reasons is that doctors are not vaccinating children properly, which shifts the blame from defective and ineffective vaccines to uncaring parents and doctors, an unlikely supposition.

Five to 25 children of every 100 vaccinated with it may be partially or even totally unprotected against the diseases. They may still develop them or an atypical form, which will make it difficult for your doctor to diagnose them. If he says your child has the measles, do not insist "it's impossible, since Teddy was vaccinated." He may be right.

The goal of the rubella vaccine, the "R" in MMR, is not to prevent children from catching German measles, a benign illness, but to prevent women from getting it during pregnancy, since it wreaks havoc on fetuses under three months of age. Partial vaccination or total failure is a serious problem, and women who intend to have children should be tested to see if they are immune to the disease.

Most of the above vaccines are recommended for adults. Check the Internet (but not at the vaccine producers' sites) before rushing to get your shot, since they may not be the best for you in all instances. The logic favoring the use of vaccines is that the adverse reactions that accompany them occur less often and are milder than the symptoms of the full-blown diseases. However, rash, orchitis, arthralgia, polyneuritis, febrile convulsions and encephalitis are among the adverse reactions reported, and they do not just sound unpleasant.

As I mentioned above, there are many vaccines available today, with more on the way. Whether they are necessary is still being debated in medical circles. The flu vaccine used to be given only in specific cases, such as to patients over age 65 or to younger people with serious health problems who might not survive the disease. This was the recommendation in an old PDR I used to refer to when I was in practice. Over the years the recommendation has grown to include everyone still breathing, irrespective of his age.

I do not believe children and healthy young adults should get the flu or Covid vaccines. People over 65 should consider Pneumovax, which is effective against pneumonia, the leading cause of death in the elderly and the chronically ill.

Like MMR, the flu vaccine does not guarantee you won't catch the illness. It is composed of viruses that have been on a rampage elsewhere in the world, and which the Public Health Service presumes have infected a boat person rowing in your direction. If his boat sinks, or the virus changes certain traits, the vaccine is useless, but its side effects may occur, and these can be far worse than the flu.

In 1976, a campaign was begun to vaccinate the entire population of the United States because the health department feared an influenza pandemic was imminent. Unfortunately, the A/New Jersey/1976/H1N1 vaccine, also known as the "swine flu" vaccine, was linked to the development of Guillain-Barré syndrome, a serious, sometimes fatal neurological disease, and the program was stopped.

In 2019 we saw a similar campaign with what I refer to as the "Covid-19 Scamdemic." The authorized but unapproved, untested vaccine that neither protects you from catching ~~the flu~~ Covid, nor from transmitting it, was forced upon the world in violation of numerous international codes, including the Nuremberg Code, and is known to be associated with serious and too often fatal side-effects. Heart attacks in young children is among the latter. Articles explaining my opinion of this situation can be found at https://gwtguide.substack.com/

Please do not begin anew a series of vaccinations simply because you lost your immunization card. The concept of vaccinations as a safe preventive medicine has been a source of debate since Jenner discovered his against smallpox, and continues today as the disaster of the Covid vaccination unfolds.

William White voiced his opinion in 1885 in the *Fallacies and Delusions of the Medical Profession* I referred to in a prior chapter:

William White, author of "Story of A Great Delusion:" "The vaccination law is unnecessary, unequal, cruel and immoral. Unnecessary, in that it has never saved a life, while it has destroyed many; unequal, in that the rich can defy it with a light heart, while it crushes the poor into an abhorred compliance; cruel, in that, falling on the poor, where it strikes it leaves either a broken fortune or a broken heart; immoral, in that where it succeeds it leaves a broken conscience."

Until this point, it has been easy to decide how to protect your health, but now comes the maze. There are no set programs about adult preventive medicine, and, therefore, you need to discuss your individual needs with your doctor.

As you age, you will fall ill with your personal illness, often rooted in your family history. This makes standardized testing for everyone impractical. For example, a yearly electrocardiogram (ECG) will not diagnose cancer of the pancreas, a disease that has mercilessly devastated one prominent American's family, and often kills within six months after its diagnosed.

If you are middle-aged, male, sedentary, obese, a heavy drinker and smoker, and suspect your heart might not be as healthy as you'd like, a routine ECG is of limited value. Even if it suggests your coronary arteries are diseased, it will not cure your bad habits nor prevent a heart attack.

So, if this is your case, since you're abusing your body, what would you like us doctors to do about your abnormal ECG? Fill you with medication to prevent what is impossible to prevent with medication? Put you on the waiting list for a future heart-lung transplant? Erase your name in the organ donor rolls?

If the only purpose of a routine ECG in an asymptomatic adult is to warn him of the possibility of a future heart attack, then let me clear the air now. To you readers who are fat, flabby, flatulent, and over forty, especially if you drink, smoke and snort cocaine, Beware! You are in danger of suffering a heart attack unless you change your life-styles *immediately*! You may now send *me* the $400.00 you saved on your cardiology work-up, and I will give it to my favorite charity where it will do some good.

Television, radio programs and magazines on newsstands have commented on the negative effects of easy living on the coronaries, and if you have not learned to direct your fate by age f44, shades of Tiberius, it is unlikely you ever will!

The ECG does serve a function, however, and you

should have one performed when you are young and store it in a safe place until you need to compare it to the one you'll get when you have chest pain and think you're having a heart attack. If the two match, it is unlikely your symptoms have anything to do with your heart. This early ECG is important if it is abnormal but you are not having symptoms, since many people have abnormal hearts on paper, yet live full, normal lives. You do not want your doctor to treat you for a 40 year-old "abnormality" he is misinterpreting as a recent disease.

Not all diseases are hereditary, but a significant problem arises when you learn your mother has Huntington's Chorea, a severe degenerative disease of the nervous system. Even though this disease and others like it carry a heavy psychological burden, not everyone wants to know his fate in these cases. If such a problem runs in your family, even if you do not want to undergo an examination that may cast a negative cloud over your future, genetic counseling may help future generations of your family. You should strongly consider it.

A history of one of the more common diseases, such as diabetes or hypertension on both family sides, should also raise suspicions. If this is your case, you should have periodic, inexpensive evaluations, not to prevent these diseases, but to begin treatment when and if it becomes necessary. Often these diseases arise because of obesity, smoking, drinking, and stress.

When I was in private practice I let my patients order certain examinations at their discretion, such as blood sugar levels, pregnancy testing, and blood pressure readings. They paid for their examinations but not for the office visit. Those who used the service knew about their diseases, or their family history of those diseases, and the reduced cost and easy access encouraged those with little money but sound concerns to seek attention sooner than they would had they had to pay for the office visit as well as the tests. I reviewed all the results and personally discussed those that were abnormal with the patient.

You may not be able to convince your doctor of this idea, but it does not hurt to ask. If he agrees, you might even ask him to include some of the more common infectious illnesses, such as strep throat and bladder infections, in the list. His nurse could perform a throat or urine culture, and if the results showed a bacterial infection, you would pay for it and the office visit. If not, you would pay just the laboratory fee.

You'll find resistance to the suggestion, but I proposed this idea many years ago in an international medical journal, and some doctors have taken up on it. "Drop-in" laboratories now exist in Anchorage, Alaska and in other places. With a little effort, you might be able to persuade your doctor to be the first in your town to offer such a service to his patients. It would benefit you both.

Now then, if you still wish to enter the wild world of the routine physical, even though its primary function is to maintain your doctor's routine bank deposit and not your health, you should know what may happen to you.

You will undergo the same history and physical examinations I described in an earlier chapter, but now they should be more broad-based and detailed, because this time you are convinced you are healthy. When you request a routine physical you do not say, "I have a headache and blurry vision," thereby telling your doctor where to look, but you challenge, "I've never felt better in my life, Doc. Prove me wrong!"

If your doctor is less thorough than when you were ill, your routine physical will degenerate into nothing more than: "Yup, you look great. Let's just run a few tests to be sure."

An exotic example of a problem arising from an incomplete history during a routine physical is that of Salome from Tonga, the land of the metal postage stamps, whose doctors had treated her repeatedly for a venereal disease based on her laboratory results. Unfortunately, they had overlooked the fact that in her country a non-sexually transmittable disease, Yaws, which tests like its more disreputable sister, Syphilis, is rampant. A letter I gave her will prevent further injections of penicillin and backroom tittering, but her case clearly shows that your doctor must question you before he orders any tests, and especially before he misinterprets them and treats you unnecessarily.

There are many gray areas in the routine physical, either because your doctor performs or interprets certain tests haphazardly, or more importantly, because he omits them because of false modesty. Knowing a few of them may be of help:

1. Blood pressure check. No physical is complete without it, but no other test wreaks more havoc than this does. It will be high at the time of your examination if you are nervous about the thought of having high blood pressure. Medical literature reports that in apprehensive people, the systolic (maximum) value may be 27 millimeters of mercury higher in the doctor's office than in friendly surroundings. Misdiagnosis and unnecessary treatment follow when a doctor decides from a single, high reading you are hypertensive, and immediately starts therapy.

People with proven high blood pressure should lower it to avoid problems such as kidney failure and stroke in later life, but medical journals now report more patients die from their medications than from their disease.

If your pressure is high during your visit, especially if you know it has been normal in the past, refuse treatment until you have had it measured on at least three other occasions when you are relaxed in comfortable surroundings. Having a friend measure it in your home would be ideal. Consider therapy only if your pressure is repeatedly high, since normal blood pressure will increase to abnormal levels when you are nervous, angry, or in pain. You do not need to treat these transitory elevations.

There are also other reasons for transient hypertension. During sexual intercourse, for example, your systolic pressure can easily exceed 200 millimeters of mercury. This is why men who have had heart attacks should not have sex with their young mistresses who will raise their pressure much more than their spouses of 40 years. A professional weight lifter, at the moment of the lift, can raise his pressure to over 300 millimeters of mercury.

Medical literature suggests you have your blood pressure checked at least once every two years, more often if it is high.

2. After age 50, I advise a yearly rectal examination to check for blood in your stool, since its presence may signal something potentially serious is growing in your intestine. You do not need routine X-rays of your intestinal tract if you have no symptoms and the exam is negative. The literature also suggests you get a colonoscopy every ten years, (a flexible tube with a camera on the end is passed through your rectum into your colon), or a double contrast barium enema. Neither of these examinations is fun.

Not every society agrees with this particular examination, and in my years in practice in Italy, males thought I was homosexual when I suggested it, and females associated it with battery. If you think the same way, modernize your thinking or stay out of your doctor's office, as an examination without this is incomplete.

A check of the prostate (found only in the male, for

you non-anatomists) is recommended every ten years, and can be done while the rectal examination is being performed. Doctors often order the prostate-specific antigen (PSA), but it doesn't necessarily mean you have cancer if it's high since. A fact to ponder: most men will have prostate cancer by they time they are 80 years old, but few will die from it. At that age men should not even be tested for the disease. Treatment of prostate cancer in a younger man is hotly discussed since it can be worse than the disease.

3. An important part of any examination is the palpation of breasts in the female and of the testicles in the male, again a font of embarrassment in certain individuals. A doctor is rarely the first to diagnose tumors of the external reproductive organs, since patients themselves usually discover them while bathing or engaging in sexual play. Since these tumors often respond favorably to therapy in the early stages, waiting for your doctor to examine those organs every now and then is not advisable, and you should perform this examination yourself monthly.

I don't recommend daily palpation for medical purposes, since you'll never notice a change in the size of a cancerous lump over a twenty-four-hour period. If you don't believe me, palpate a tomato on its vine every day. You are less likely to notice its increase in size than if you check it every other week.

Charts explaining breast examination technique are available in your doctor's office or your local health department. You should examine your breasts after your period since cysts under hormonal control are common. If your breasts were normal last month and now you have a large, tender, lump in one, the odds are it is a cyst. Cancer does not grow that fast and is not painful that soon, which is unfortunate. If it were painful in its early stages, it would be much easier to find and cure. A cyst will usually disappear after your period. If it lasts for a month or two, have it checked.

Mammograms are another source of heated debate for different reasons. The American Cancer Society recommends women over 40 have one every year. Since some breast tumors will disappear on their own, these X-rays often result in unnecessary repeat studies and biopsies. The literature suggests 2,500 women in their forties would need regular mammograms to extend just one life. Since that life may be yours, I'll let you decide on your course of action.

A pelvic examination is done to determine the size and shape of your internal reproductive organs. This exam does not necessarily include a Pap test, described below, and is recommended every three years in women under 40, yearly in those over 40. Ovaries should not be palpable after menopause, and if one is, it may be due to cancer.

This is the theory, but in reality the bimanual pelvic examination is unsatisfactory. The normal ovary is a one-inch long mass of tissue buried deep in the pelvis, which a doctor tries to palpate between his finger inside your vagina and his other hand over your lower abdomen. The likelihood of correctly determining the size of your ovary falls in proportion to the increasing thickness of your abdominal wall. If you place a Ping-Pong ball under a sheet, you will have no trouble in determining its shape and size. If you place it under seventeen quilts....

Examples of difficulties determining organ size are the often told story of the obese woman who did not know she was pregnant until she delivered her baby, and the tale of the nurse who had a 20 pound ovarian cyst removed surgically three months after her "normal" pelvic exam.

If you're a sylph in *Cosmopolitan* magazine, your doctor will have little trouble finding a mass in your belly, but if you are a Suma wrestler, I would not be optimistic about the validity of the examination.

Doctors will order ultrasound scans when they want to know the exact sizes of the organs, but this is not foolproof either. I once examined a patient who had had a normal pelvic examination and a normal ultrasound of her ovaries six months earlier. When I examined her, she had two five inch diameter tumors in her pelvis, which were diagnosed as ovarian cancers at surgery. Fortunately, they had not spread out of her pelvis and further therapy has seemingly cured her.

Ovarian cancer is virulent and unpleasant. Do not ignore low abdominal pain and pressure even if your pap and pelvic examinations a few months earlier were normal.

An aside: you can discover your doctor's leisure habits from his explanation of his findings after your examination. If he describes your lumps and bumps as "large as a potato, small as a cherry," he has a green thumb. If he says they are as "big as a baseball," or "like a golf ball," he is sport's minded. If he uses inches or centimeters, he is simply being professional.

The Pap smear detects cancer of the cervix. Its problems include errors in interpretation and the frequency with which it should be performed. There are those who recommend a woman get it every six months, but since it takes five years for cancer of the cervix to develop once the process has started, performing the Pap smear semiannually in a patient with a previously normal test is unnecessary. A more rational schedule would be to repeat it every three years if the first two tests were normal, and more often if you are taking birth control pills or have symptoms of pelvic disease.

If you do have it done, ask to see the written report. I had a patient who was told by an automated telephone report from her gynecologist's office, that her HPV (human papillomavirus which causes genital warts and cervical cancer) and Pap tests were normal. Since she had specifically refused the HPV test and was concerned she might have been billed for it, she asked for a copy of her report. Across its middle someone had written, "neg Pap, neg HPV," yet the report itself stated clearly, "no HPV testing was performed."

She wondered why she had even had the test done after reading the warning on the report, "(the Pap smear) is not a diagnostic procedure and should not be used as the sole means of detecting cervical cancer. Both false positive and false-negative reports do occur." She was also critical of the doctor who did not even have the courtesy to have a live employee call her with her report.

4. Routine physicals usually include routine blood tests. A blood count will tell you how many red and white cells you have in circulation, but misinterpretation of even this simple test can create problems. A doctor may sometimes tell his tired, pale patient in bad spirits, she is grumpy because she is anemic, even though the real culprits are overwork, depression, and natural skin coloring. The iron pills he'll prescribe won't cure any of those causes.

Other tests performed as a panel often create panic when their results deviate from the norm. If most of the 20 or 30 tests in you panel are abnormal, then so are you. If only one test is, as a rule the machine is ill. Have the test repeated if you are concerned, but do not begin therapy before you do.

"Do you have high cholesterol?" is a question often asked at parties, right after, "What is your astrological sign?" If you do, a suitable diet will lower it safely by 10% to 15%. Medications will decrease the level another 10% but not without consequences, and they will *not* prevent heart attacks.

In a report a few years ago of two groups of patients with high cholesterol, there were 29 deaths in the one treated with a pill and none in the group treated with diet alone. This medication, clofibrate, has been associated with an increased risk of gallstones and an increased risk of tumors in humans, but I think rats are safe from this one. I know you will consult your PDR and the Internet before starting a long-term therapy with this or any of the other cholesterol lowering drugs that are advertised on TV.

One last important point: if you ride the laboratory conveyor belt, personally review your test results in your doctor's office, or ask him to send you a copy of them. *Under no condition* accept his promise, "if you do not hear from me, it means everything is OK." I once examined a patient with uterine cancer who told me she had been "cured by surgery," because her Pap test a year earlier was negative. She had not asked to see her report. When I saw it, it was compatible with invasive cancer. Her doctor never got back to her, but he had told her not to worry if she did not hear from him in a week. The unfortunate woman stopped worrying a long while ago.

Before entering a doctor's office for any purpose, particularly for preventive medicine purposes, remember the following:

Apart from vitamin C (this is *not* cocaine), there is no harmless medication or infallible treatment. This includes aspirin, Tylenol, vaccinations, and all medical or surgical procedures.

Therapy and prevention are a mixture of benefits and side effects. If you understand and choose to accept them, you share responsibility for all their effects, good and bad, with those who supply or administer them.

The best advice I can give you for a long life, after selective vaccination, is choose healthy parents, avoid bad habits, and keep a watchful eye on your environment, as your city health department is more important to you than your doctor in preventing disease.

EPILOGUE: WOULDN'T IT BE NICE IF...?

Medicine is a business, and if your idea of it as a profession whose primary goal is to relieve your suffering, you are mistaken. Doctors and their staffs have reduced us to disembodied organs ("There's a cataract in the waiting room, Doctor."), and insurance companies, HMOs and the government have reduced us even further. To them we and our diseases are nothing more than numbers (Patient 89505487A has 90050).

Employees from these organizations decide from their offices miles away from our bedsides which treatment is permissible and which is not, as well the maximum time they will allow us to recover from our illnesses before they stop payment.

Bureaucratic whining has become more complex over the years, and the solutions to the problems it has spawned are limited to playing catch-up. But while I was pondering the situation, and maybe even dreaming a little, the following thought came to my mind: Just once, wouldn't it be nice to hear the doctor say:

"I have no idea what your problem is, Mr. Smith. Let me send you to someone who might, and I won't charge you for this office visit."

"Only one of the 53 tests I ordered for you was positive. I am going to refund the costs of the unnecessary exams."

"You didn't need a hysterectomy after all Mrs. Smith. The hospital and I are going to refund you your money."

"It is important to keep a close watch on your blood pressure. All these office visits are expensive, but now that it has returned to normal, if you have it checked at least every three months, my staff will check it at no charge."

"Although the flu shot serves no purpose in many patients, we do not charge for it in this office because the state gives us the vaccine for free."

"If you have recovered from your problem in seven days, you do not need to return to this office."

"This is my home telephone number, Mr. Jones. Call me any time, day or night, you feel you need my services."

"You do not need an injection to cure your problem. Giving you one will only make me richer."

"We have an opening in ten minutes, Mr. Green. In this office we feel you should be seen as soon as you do."

"I'm sorry you had to wait so long. Please accept my apologies and a 50% discount on your charges for today."

"Before you leave, do you have any further questions about your illness or the medicine I've prescribed for you?"

"This is Dr. Baker, Mr. Peters. I hope I'm not disturbing you. I'm calling to see how you are getting along."

BIBLIOGRAPHY

Andrews Raymond C. "More on serve-yourself clinical laboratories." New England Journal of Medicine, 13 Nov. 1980; **303**:1183.

- - -. "Laetrile." New England Journal of Medicine, 8 July 1982; **307**:119.

- - -. "Doctor's Inside View of Socialized Medicine." Bakersfield Californian, 29 Oct. 1978.

- - -. "Emergency Room Abuses Related." Bakersfield Californian, 24 Dec. 1978.

- - -. "High Medical Cost of Emergency Care." Bakersfield Californian, 22 Apr. 1979.

- - -. "The Spiraling Costs of Medical Care." Bakersfield Californian, 3 June 1979.

- - -. "Foreign socialized medicine vs. U.S. health care system." Bakersfield Californian, 8 Nov. 1981.

- - -. "Which is better: pay-as-you-go medicine or socialized medicine?" The Record, 11 Oct. 1981.

Angel JE (publisher). Physicians' Desk Reference, 38th ed. Medical Economics Company, 1984.

Barnhart ER (publisher). Physicians' Desk Reference for Nonprescription Drugs, 5th ed. Medical Economics Company, 1984.

Poggiolini D (editor). *Clofibrato e suoi derivati*. Bollettino d'informazione sui Farmaci, Nov. 1988; **11**:2.

Crossland J. Lewis's Pharmacology. E & S Livingstone, 1970.

Ebert R, Enders J, et al: Letter. <u>New York Times,</u> 10 Jan. 1977.

Garrison FH. <u>History of Medicine</u>. W.B. Saunders Company, 1929.

Guthrie DJ et al. "History of Medicine." Pages 823-841 in: <u>The New Encyclopedia Britannica</u>. Chicago, vol. 11, 1981.

Johnson GT (editor). "Personal Health Maintenance-Part I." <u>Harvard Medical School Health Letter</u>, Mar. 1977; **2**:1.

- - -. "Personal Health Maintenance-Part II." <u>Harvard Medical School Health Letter</u>, Apr. 1977; **2**:2-3.

Krupp MA, Chatton MJ (editors). <u>Current Medical Diagnosis & Treatment</u>. Lange Medical Publications, 1983.

Laennec RTH. <u>A Treatise on the Diseases of the Chest</u>. Underwood, 1821. (Reprinted for The Classics of Medicine Library, Gryphon Editions, Ltd., 1979.)

Lewin et al. Conference: Industry analysis. <u>Studies in the comparative performance of investor-owned and not-for-profit hospitals</u>. Washington, D.C., vol. 1, 1981.

- - -. Conference: The comparative economic performance of a matched sample of investor-owned and not-for-profit hospitals. <u>Studies in the comparative performance of investor-owned and not-for-profit hospitals</u>. Washington, D.C., vol. 4, 1981.

Manson JM. 1986. Teratogenicity. Cassarett and Doull's <u>Toxicology: The Basic Science of Poisons.</u> Third Edition. Pages 195-220. New York: MacMillan Publishing Co.

Nante G. "*Di ospedale si può morire*." <u>Il Medico d'Italia,</u> 1986, **69**:9.

"Nearly all are wrong." Parade Magazine, 15 July 1984.

Osler W. <u>The Principles and Practice of Medicine</u>. D.

Appleton and Company, 1892. (Reprinted for The Classics of Medicine Library, Gryphon Editions, Ltd., 1978.)

Pattison RV, Katz HM. "Investor-owned and not-for-profit hospitals." New England Journal of Medicine 1983, **309**:347-53.

Platt R. "Cost containment – another view." New England Journal of Medicine, 1983; **309**:726-30.

Relman AS. "Investor-owned hospitals and health care costs." New England Journal of Medicine, 1983; **309**:370-72.

Rose P. "'Addict' patients threaten action on tranquilliser (sic)." Daily Mail (London), 16 Dec. 1987; 2.

Ross, Alexander M. "Fallacies and Delusions of the Medical Profession." Toronto, 1888.

Rubenstein E, Federman DD (editors). "Gram-Positive Cocci." Scientific American Medicine. New York, vol. 2, 1979.

Schorr B. "Laboratory Kickbacks to Doctors Persist Despite Federal and State Investigations." The Wall Street Journal, 26 Sept. 1978; 40.

Shapiro, Scott (Fenton Communications), Loughran, Sara (HealthGades). "In Hospital Deaths from Medical Errors at 195,000 per Year USA." Medical News Today, 9 Aug. 2004.

Smithels RW and Newman CG. 1992. J. Med. Genet. 29(10):716-723.

Tierney, Jr. LM, McPhee SJ, Papadakis MA (editors). Current Medical Diagnosis & Treatment. Lange Medical Publications, 1995.

Vickery DM, Fries JF. Take Care of Yourself, A Consumer's Guide to Medical Care. Addison-Wesley Publishing Company, 1984.

The Author

Raymond C. Andrews is an American born physician who graduated from the University of Bologna Medical School in Italy in 1970. After training in general surgery, neurosurgery, and aerospace medicine, he accepted the position as an emergency room director in a New Jersey hospital.

In the late 1970s he entered private practice in California and later wrote a popular series of articles on health care for the Bakersfield *Californian*. Other articles and comments of his have appeared in the *New England Journal of Medicine*, the *Bergen Record*, and *Private Practice*. While in practice he developed "Drop-in-Laboratory Services" to make access to medical care easier and less costly for the migrant workers that comprised much his patients.

Lured back to Italy by medieval castles and the opera at *La Scala* in 1984, Dr. Andrews worked ten years for the state health system. He was the first physician to participate in the newly established Italian emergency hot-line system.

After twenty-five years of medical practice on two continents, and with the regrettable certainty that patient care has taken a back seat to bureaucracy and to the questionable tactics of some of his colleagues both here and abroad, in 1995 he accepted a position with the United States Public Health Service and was a director of a Navajo clinic on their reservation in northeastern Arizona. He was also director of the clinic's Emergency Medical Services, and a director of the National Native American Emergency Medical Services Association.

Dr. Andrews is retired and passes his time writing, building model ships, and driving his modified Jeep and camper in the Arizona desert